AMPossible

AMPossible

Real-World Solutions to Help Amputees Accomplish the Impossible

Jeffrey Allen Mangus

ROWMAN & LITTLEFIELD

Lanham · Boulder · New York · London

Published by Rowman & Littlefield
An imprint of The Rowman & Littlefield Publishing Group, Inc.
4501 Forbes Boulevard, Suite 200, Lanham, Maryland 20706
www.rowman.com

6 Tinworth Street, London SE11 5AL, United Kingdom

British Library Cataloguing in Publication Information Available

Library of Congress Cataloging-in-Publication Data

Names: Mangus, Jeffrey Allen, 1966- author.
Title: AMPossible : real-world solutions to help amputees accomplish the impossible / Jeffrey Allen Mangus.
Description: Lanham : Rowman & Littlefield, [2021] | Includes bibliographical references and index.
Identifiers: LCCN 2020054140 (print) | LCCN 2020054141 (ebook) | ISBN 9781538141878 (cloth) | ISBN 9781538141885 (epub)
Subjects: LCSH: Amputees—Rehabilitation. | Amputees—Psychology.
Classification: LCC RD756 .M319 2021 (print) | LCC RD756 (ebook) | DDC 617.5/8—dc23
LC record available at https://lccn.loc.gov/2020054140
LC ebook record available at https://lccn.loc.gov/2020054141

I want to dedicate this book to my wife, Kelly, who stood beside me, lifted me up from the bottom, carried me, and showed the world the true meaning of "For Better or For Worse." I love you with all my heart and soul. Thank you for never quitting and always seeing the best in me.

This book is also dedicated to our five children: Brady, Ryann, Gabby, Jacob, and Sophie, along with Thaddaeus, Katie, and Allison and my grandkids Elora Grace and Liesel Sue.

I cannot forget my late friend John Gillenwater, who was there for me and my family through every painful step of my limb loss journey, unconditionally. I love and miss you, my brother. RIP

Lastly, I dedicate this book to my mom and dad, Irene and Fred, and my sister, Dianna, who have always been there through it all. I love all of you very much.

Contents

Part V. Regaining Your Independence and Life

Part VI. Making the Impossible Possible

Preface

My Limb Loss Story

"*We* have to take you to surgery now!" the doctor shouted as my fever raged and cold, clammy sweat poured out of me. Around me, nurses and medical staff swarmed as I struggled to breathe. My engorged left foot was a sickening green, oozing with infection, and little did I know that my life was hanging in the balance. Only hours before I had unraveled the bandage from my left foot to find it swollen three times its usual size and green as a dying weed. Even as I stared at my foot, I didn't realize that the day I had planned was shaping up to be a nightmare that would change the course of my life.

For three years I had been battling continuous wounds on my feet as a result of diabetes. At this point I was used to the normal routine of going to the hospital, getting treatment, bandaged, and being sent home. Even as I hobbled to the car, shoeless, foot engorged, I thought to myself, *They will examine me, clean my wound, give me a strong anti-biotic, and send me on my way.* I was confident that the doctors would bandage me up, stick me in the ass with antibiotics, and send me home to fight another day.

This time I was dead wrong.

When I pulled into the parking lot of the hospital the air had a strange stillness; everything was seemingly dark and gray. As I turned off the car's engine, I sat, remaining completely still. Surrounding me was a feeling I could not ignore—a strong presence signaling every ounce of my being that things were about to change. Not knowing and scared, I suddenly felt the need to squeeze every second I could, and I didn't know why. I took a deep breath, embraced the moment while listening to the whisper of the stillness. As I made my way to the emergency room, a soft voice told me, *"It will be okay."* A cascading peace washed over me as the doors of the emergency room closed behind me. Little did I know that in a few short hours that walk would be the last I would ever take—with my own two legs.

Acknowledgments

$\mathcal{I}$ would like to acknowledge Mr. Warren Tuttle, president of Tuttle Innovation and president of the United Inventors Association for being instrumental in helping me start my writing career, believing in me, and being my dear and close friend every step of the way.

Thank you to my agent, Gary Krebs, for believing in me and this book from the very beginning. Thank you for all the help and guidance throughout. I could not have done it without you.

I want to acknowledge and deeply thank my editor, Suzanne Staszak-Silva, for her belief in this book project, guidance, and making the writing process one I'll never forget.

I

FACING THE AMPUTATION

Introduction

From every trial in life, there is a wound, and from every wound, there is a scar. And from every scar, there is a story that says, I survived.

— Unknown

*T*hree years prior to that walk through the emergency room doors, the little toe on my left foot was amputated due to a wound that never healed. That amputation was my first, and I admit, before the toe loss, I did not effectively manage my diabetes. I am a type 2 diabetic. I ignored the signs and lived haphazardly with vast amounts of stress, terrible food choices, and worst of all—no sleep. I was a walking time bomb. It was utterly my fault, and I had no one else to blame. After an immense amount of soul-searching, I decided that losing a toe was the last straw. I had to make drastic changes in my life. I attacked my health and diabetes head-on and began taking care of myself. Within six months, after eating an all-vegetable (no meat) diet and following strict diabetic management, I dropped my A1C from 18 to 7.1. It was a vast improvement; however, this is when things began to unravel.

Even though I was eating healthy and following a strict diabetic management plan, my left foot would not completely heal. The doctors were baffled, yet healing efforts went on for two years with extensive wound care treatments. It was exhausting, frustrating, and tiresome, yet despite all efforts, the nickel-sized wound remained. I never realized that I was playing Russian roulette with my life by going in and out of the wound care facility daily. The wound clinic was a cesspool of germs with bacteria hidden in the smallest and darkest of places, and the odds eventually became too great.

I lost the game.

As my foot became severely infected, I still never thought the worst. I had a fever and chills and believed I was coming down with the flu, but I grew weaker, lethargic, and eventually sepsis set in and took over my body. Everything seemed to be slowly shutting down as my kidneys began to fail, and my heart struggled to beat. My body was struggling from the massive infection in my foot. My brain and organs were not receiving enough blood to function, turning my situation critical. I didn't have a choice when my surgeon emphatically announced that I needed to go to surgery if I wanted to live. My world was spiraling, fading, and still I never dreamed that I was facing losing my limb—and even death.

I was fifty-one years old on November 29, 2017, when my world crashed to a grinding halt, changing it forever. My left foot was inflamed with infection, and in this fleeting, horrifying moment, I was now faced with the inevitable choice of losing it or risking pending death. Doctors and nurses scrambled and rushed me immediately into surgery. (The amputation on that foot was the first of three major operations.) I woke to the sight of the entire top of my left foot, including all muscles, tendons, and ligaments, removed. My heart sank at the spectacle; my foot torn to shreds, damaged beyond healing. I now faced a life-altering decision—to amputate or never walk normally again.

I made the heart-wrenching decision to amputate my foot and salvage what I thought was left of my life. However, things would not be that easy. During the second operation—the removal of my foot—the surgeons discovered a massive infection throughout my leg and in the tibia bone. This forced them to stop the amputation, cut my leg straight down "guillotine style," take a sample of the infected area, and analyze it.

Then I had to wait.

Waiting for the results was pure agony as I had to lie with my leg elevated and in horrifying and gripping pain. To make matters even worse, for an entire week and a half, I waited in angst and agony, unknowing and unsure of how much more of my left leg I was going to lose. Finally, the results came back showing the infection was no longer life-threatening, but it had spread higher than predicted within my bone.

Things looked grim—I now faced losing even more of my leg.

The surgeons decided precisely how much more of my leg they had to take, and they amputated my left leg just below the knee.

I wrote this book after realizing firsthand the drastic need to explain amputation and the life-changing dose of reality that it brings. For me, this lack of knowledge was a major frustration because the treatment I received during my limb loss was a bizarre, unanswered event riddled with complacency and massive mistakes. What I found most disturbing was the sickening apathy, lack of emotional connection, and human compassion among some (not all) of my immediate health-care team. There were shining stars among the team (you know who you are). Still, most of the critical questions I had, sadly, went unanswered. Even worse, certain treatments and therapies that I needed were oddly never put into place. Not knowing what to expect was one of the hardest aspects of my recovery. During the darkest time of my life, my wife and I desperately needed answers about life, how to move forward, how to cope, and how to even try to live again.

But the answers did not come.

During the early days of my recovery I needed a go-to resource that would provide real-world guidance and understanding of what was truly happening. Losing my left leg saved my life, yet what I experienced post-surgery with the health-care team, treating my amputation as merely routine, was confusing, frustrating, and unsettling. I recognized that people don't lose limbs every day, and when it happens quickly life changes drastically, bringing many pending and important questions to mind. My intent with this book is to provide you those answers. I understand that right now everything may seem traumatic, dark, hopeless, magnified, and out of control. It did for me. It was frightening as both my wife and I faced the unknown and didn't understand what to do or where our lives were headed. Everything around me was spinning, and I had so many questions, but it seemed no one would answer them. Still, no matter how hard I tried, it seemed no one was listening. So I sought to write a book that would answer those pertinent and personal questions, shed light on those subjects not talked about, and, most of all, provide much-needed guidance, compassion, and understanding, and instill hope during this traumatic time.

Amputation is one of the hardest, most emotional, and fearful things a person will ever have to experience. Every amputation shocks the patient's very existence to their core in ways they never expected, so this book is written for all amputees across the globe, young and old, novice or experienced, with the intent to help and guide you through this difficult journey. Whether you are an upper extremity or lower extremity amputee, I hope that you will find in this book the answers that will help you live a healthy and beautiful life.

I understand some portions of the book may not pertain to all amputees, yet I encourage you to read the entire book and share it with your family and friends. My goal is for you and your family to learn everything about living as an amputee from a real, hands-on, firsthand point of view. I have strived to leave no stone unturned and talk about pertinent subjects including pain management, phantom pains, depression, anxiety, prosthetics, sexuality, rejection, acceptance, driving, physical therapy, and handling and coping with your emotions. I have poured my heart into this book to help you get the best chance at living a great life as an amputee and not a view from the cheap seats.

During this traumatic time, fear can grip everyone in your circle as they experience your limb loss alongside you. Use and share this book as a go-to guide for everyone in your life. Your surrounding people play an integral role in your recovery, and they should know what to expect in their lives as well with your amputation. My goal for your family is to provide helpful and insightful answers to their tough questions while offering potential solutions to everyday problems experienced by a new amputee.

Amputation affects everything from how you function at home, at work, and in the world. It also affects finances, careers, and relationships with spouses, family, friends, and coworkers. If you are a lower limb amputee, your ability to move around, walk, and stand on two feet will be drastically altered. If you are an upper extremity amputee, everything you do with your arms, fingers, and hands will be dramatically changed. And if this reality isn't hard enough, after you regain the physical aspects of your life, you will have to address the difficult emotional recovery. The emotional recovery after limb loss can often be harder than the physical challenges. What I have learned on my limb loss journey is that amputation, as a way of life, will take perseverance, strength, understanding, attitude, and, most of all, allowing yourself time to heal.

Limb loss is devastating in more ways than just physically losing your limb/s. Recovery is fraught with difficult mental challenges where you may feel as if you have completely lost yourself. I want you to use this book as a guide to find yourself, get back to center, and help you retain the life you once had. You can do it, yet make no mistake, it will be one of the hardest challenges you will ever face. The key is to work hard and believe in yourself to replenish your life and put it all back into place. Everything, from this moment on, is up to you.

When I first lost my left leg, everything seemed distorted, and I was an emotional train wreck filled with anger, confusion, and overwhelming feelings of being cheated out of my life. At first I could not see the gifts of the new life before me because they were hidden behind a wall of hurt, pain, and sadness. Yet, through it all, these gifts have given me a sense of being, self-worth, and a different trajectory, guiding my life's purpose to help others live prosperous, healthy, and more vibrant lives.

Without enduring the hurt, the struggle, and the pain, I never would have found the strength and courage necessary to fight the good fight and hold the line to be here today. As I fought, screamed, cried, and struggled through my recovery, I discovered a newfound inner strength and uncovered a selfless spirit ready and willing to uplift and support others through honest actions and reactions to my limb loss. And I ultimately hope that you will, too.

Today, if someone were to ask me to trade my life as an amputee for another brand-new life with all my limbs, my answer would be a resounding NO. Yet in the minutes and days after my limb loss, there wasn't a soul on earth who could convince me that I would ever say those words. Still, my limb loss has allowed me to conquer some of the hardest challenges of my life and, along the way, discover the strong-willed man—the real person—I was inside. I wouldn't trade that experience for anything.

You, as an amputee, will now face significant complexities and hardships, and I know you have the power within to overcome these newfound challenges set before you. You may not see it now, but I know that you possess the strength to survive the immense change, grief, and loss. I believe you have it inside of you to fight through the intense pain and deep-rooted, entangled emotions to reach a full, abundant life once again.

Lastly, I hope that this book will allow you to rise above the fray during your limb loss journey. This book's sole purpose is to give you a foundational reminder that your new life has inherent value, and everything you have and more is worthy of fighting to get back. Remember, your life is worthwhile and priceless, and even though it's now missing a part, you still have much to offer—more now than ever before. Take a deep breath and do everything within your power to work, fight, and push through to live the fullest life imaginable. Do everything possible to change your life, and you may be surprised that through your courage and tenacity, you may change others. I sincerely hope you do.

— Jeffrey A. Mangus

II

BEFORE YOUR AMPUTATION

• 1 •

Causes for Amputation

You can be afraid and still strong, still fearless, and in-
domitable. You can be afraid, and you can trust, and then
when you're ready, you can let go of the fear. Fear muffles
you. Let it go, and then you can live out loud again like
you're meant to.

—April White, Code of Conduct

The 1970s and 1980s were an incredible time to grow up. During that
time, I experienced many new and exciting things. However, something
I've never forgotten was a man who sat in a wheelchair on the corner of
my street—he had only one leg. Being a kid, I had never seen a missing
limb. It scared me, yet somehow captivated my attention. The man's
fake leg was made of wood and looked old, dingy, and scarred. Every
day he sat alone and silent in his wheelchair as my friends and I passed
him by on the way to school. Often, being afraid, I tried to avoid and
ignore him—yet I couldn't. I always wondered to myself, *What happened
to him? How did he lose his leg?* I told myself, *Go on, just walk over and
ask him.* My friends never seemed to notice him, but I sure did. Peer
pressure is tough, and I knew my friends would do something stupid
to me, or the old man, if I approached him, but I desperately wanted
to stop and ask him about his leg. I was curious and fascinated about
his amputation, and I never understood why. Like most kids my age I
watched old war movies and I wondered if he lost his leg like the heroes
I saw on TV, on the battlefield with guns and bombs blazing. Regrettably, I never summoned the guts to stop and ask or even talk to him.
Then one day he was gone, and I never saw him again.

11

To this day, as an amputee myself, I am reminded of this forgotten man, and now, more than ever, I regret not asking him the questions that burned inside of me. I'll never know the cause, his experience, the pain, and the hardship that he endured. When I lost my foot, thoughts of this old man came flooding back, unanswered questions about what he must have endured.

The suffering.

The struggle.

The loss.

I never knew what happened to him, but I know exactly what had happened to me. After my limb loss, I wanted to know more about the many other severe, traumatic, and unforeseen causes of amputations. According to the Amputee Coalition, among those living with limb loss, the leading causes are vascular disease (54 percent), including diabetes and peripheral arterial disease, trauma (45 percent), and cancer (less than 2 percent).[1] Whether it is caused by disease or injury, the majority derive from health-related issues stemming directly and indirectly from the following:

1. Irreparable limb injury
2. Heart attack
3. Stroke
4. Frostbite
5. Traumatic event (accident, casualty, combat)
6. Diabetes (poor management)
7. Pressure sores
8. Poor blood circulation to the limb
9. Prevention of the spreading of bone cancer
10. Blood loss control

LEADING CAUSES OF AMPUTATION

The causes of amputation can be broken down into two main categories: traumatic and nontraumatic. They're categorized as such depending on their specific causes. Injuries in the workplace (e.g., mechanical, machinery, or tool accidents), motorcycle or vehicular accidents, casualties of war (e.g., bombs, gunshots, explosions), natural (acts of God), accidents (lawnmowers, bicycles, falls), and so on, are traumatic causes. Nontraumatic causes include poor circulation, insufficient blood flow to the extremities, cancer, tumors, congenital conditions, neuropathy, infections, and wounds from diseases like diabetes.

Diabetes

Diabetes, known as the silent killer, is a severe disease of global proportions. According to the Centers for Disease Control and Prevention (CDC), diabetes affects 25.8 million Americans—that's 8.3 percent of the U.S. population. The number of amputations caused by diabetes increased by 24 percent from 1988 to 2009.[2] An excerpt from the 2017 National Diabetes Statistics Report notes an accurate point-in-time analysis[33] and provides the following information:

- Nearly one in ten Americans, 30.3 million people, have diabetes.
- Approximately one in three people, 84.1 million American adults, have prediabetes.
- More than half of newly diagnosed diabetes cases were in adults forty-five to sixty-four years old.

Diabetes and amputations stemming from it are skyrocketing. Worldwide, the diabetes epidemic is of global proportions. Annually, the CDC reports the staggering numbers of amputations in the United States for diabetics, not related to trauma. According to multiple sources, in the United States, most new amputations occur due to complications of the vascular system (blood vessels), especially from diabetes. In the United Kingdom between 2012–2016, limb loss from diabetes had risen to a staggering 7,300 per year. Of the nontraumatic amputations in the United States, 60 percent are performed on people with diabetes.[4] In 2006, about 65,700 nontraumatic lower-limb amputations were performed each year among people with diabetes. Severe forms of diabetic nerve disease are a major contributing cause of lower-extremity amputations. These numbers indicate, worldwide, that every thirty seconds a person loses a limb from diabetes.

Diabetes can result in a multitude of complications from diabetes, however not all lead to amputation. Yet many complications from diabetes progress, threaten lives, and even lead to death. They are:

- Neuropathy
- Carpal Tunnel Syndrome

- Arthritis
- High Blood Pressure
- Dental Disease
- Heart Disease

Diabetes can be considered the catalyst for the many complications leading to amputation. However, one of the most significant and problematic causes of amputation in diabetics is neuropathy, which causes numbness in the upper and lower extremities, resulting in the person not being able to detect injuries. When this happens, it can lead to unawareness and neglected care, causing the patient to be susceptible to infection, which can lead to amputation.

Peripheral Artery Disease

Peripheral artery disease (PAD) affects more than eight million Americans. It's a narrowing of the artery walls, restricting blood flow to organs and limbs, causing wounds and infections that can lead to amputations. PAD is a significant cause of cardiovascular disease, reduced mobility, limited extremity functionality, and limb loss. It often occurs in the lower extremities, causing wounds and ulcers. These critical medical conditions are treated with lower extremity amputation. PAD takes place in the arteries and causes muscle and joint fatigue and pain. Problematic issues related to PAD can go undetected and affect the blood and oxygen supply to your kidneys, stomach, intestines, arms, hands, legs, and feet.

PAD can be detected through pain in the legs or arms. It can be felt while walking or through physical exertion and goes away when the person is resting. Other signs of PAD in the lower extremities could be hair loss, smooth skin, sensitive skin, cold skin, muscle tightness or atrophy, and numbness in the legs, feet, or toes. Often, PAD goes undetected because the patient feels no pain.

Cancer

Amputation among cancer patients is rare, yet it does happen. Reports from the CDC note that among those living with limb loss, they also suffer from vascular disease (54%), including diabetes and peripheral arterial disease, trauma (45%), and cancer (less than 2%).[5] Out of the thousands of different cancers, the most prevalent leading to amputation of a limb is bone cancer, medically termed as osteosarcoma. There are only twenty thousand cases of bone cancer reported in the United States per year,[6] and they predominately occur in young adults and teens.[7] When amputation is necessary, most surgeons do their best to salvage the bone and perform what they call limb-sparing surgery. However, a surgeon could also elect to remove the cancerous bone if the cancer has spread into major blood vessels or major nerves surrounding any bone or tumor. When a surgeon chooses to amputate, they will remove the cancerous segment along with a portion of healthy tissue above and below the tumorous matter to ensure the removal of all cancer for a healthy recovery. The rates of surviving this type of bone cancer are dramatically increased when the cancerous bone is successfully removed. When bone cancer is diagnosed, amputation may be a life-saving procedure that prevents further spread of the disease.

Congenital Amputations

Congenital amputations take place in newborn babies who are born with a deformed or missing limb. Researchers have not found a specific cause for these types of disfigurements, and, fortunately, congenital amputations are one of the least common. It is rare for babies to be born in this condition, and it's estimated that one out of every two thousand babies are born with a congenital disfigurement. Yet there have been events throughout history where there were increases in babies born with birth defects. In the 1960s, a tragedy took place when pregnant women were given thalidomide. Afterward, more than ten thousand infants were born with missing limbs and other deformities.[8] Another significant event responsible for many birth defects, deformities, and missing limbs was the Chernobyl nuclear reactor explosion on April 26, 1986, in Ukraine. Afterward, more than six hundred thousand babies and children were directly affected by radiation exposure. Since then, studies have shown that children's health in that region has been deteriorating every year.

According to the Amputee Coalition, there are two main categories of limb loss in children: congenital limb deficiency and acquired amputations. A congenital limb deficiency is present at birth and can involve either the upper or lower limbs. Fortunately, multiple limb deficiencies occur rarely. Congenital deficiencies can be the complete absence of a limb, or more commonly part of the limb is missing and the remaining portion has not formed normally.[8]

War and Combat

Soldiers are elite, unsung heroes who fight to protect our freedoms and sovereignty. Throughout history soldiers have fought in wars where their injuries have included significant loss of limbs. According to historical records, on the morning of June 3, 1861, James Edgar Hangar, founder of the Hangar Clinic, was a newly enlisted private assigned to guard duty at a local farm in Philippi, West Virginia. In the first battle of the Civil War, the young Hanger ran into a barn to get his horse. A six-pound cannon ball crashed into the barn and ricocheted off a door post. The cannon ball struck Hanger in the left leg near the knee joint and then "passed through six thicknesses of two or two and a half oak plank stall partitions and partially penetrated the seventh. There its momentum was exhausted, and the ball fell in the stall." Unable to walk with his wounded leg hanging by a small part of the skin, Hanger dragged himself into the hay loft to hide. Fortunately, he was found by Union scouts several hours later. Shortly thereafter, Dr. James D. Robison of the 16th Ohio Infantry, assisted by surgeon George W. New of the 7th Indiana Infantry, performed an amputation of Hanger's leg seven inches below the hip—the first recorded amputation of the Civil War.[9]

Today, soldiers are deployed to other countries far and wide, where many experience traumatic bomb explosions or situations leaving massive injuries that can lead to loss of limbs. Injuries to soldiers that involve amputation are drastically traumatic on multiple levels, not only physically but mentally and emotionally. The mental effects of amputation have been found to have a profound and devastating impact on veterans. Even though the advancement in bodily protection and medical technology has prevented many war-time amputations, they still occur. Data from the Iraq War report that more than 1,091 traumatic combat amputations were performed. According to the 2009 United States military casualty statistics report, published by the Congressional Research Service (CRS), the amputee population in the U.S. military due to Operation Iraqi Freedom comprises 1,091 service members.[10] This number represents 85 percent of the total servicemen and -women amputations that occurred between 2001–2009. More than 50 percent of the injuries were caused by improvised explosive devices. According to the CRS, in Afghanistan, a total of 1,558 soldiers endured major limb amputations following battlefield injuries.[11] Major limb amputations include the loss of one or more limbs, losing one or more partial limbs, or losing a full or partial hand, foot, finger, or leg. Yet traumatic amputation among soldiers and veterans involves deeper scars, as most endure problematic symptoms with their mental health stability stemming from the change in life from disfigurement and limb loss. These emotional and psychological issues arise because of body image and rejection in social and work environments.

Smoking

Smoking is one of the leading causes of PAD, which is one of the main causes of amputation. Giving up smoking is an essential step in preventing PAD and amputation. Smoking tobacco products constricts your blood vessels and damages your arteries. Most associate smoking with heart attacks, stroke, and lung cancer, yet the second major cause of amputation is smoking. The harm to your vascular system caused by smoking damages blood vessels and results in irreparable disease. According to the CDC, if a person smokes one or two packs of cigarettes a day, it can lead to Buerger's disease.[12] This disease affects the body's blood vessels, constricting veins and arteries in the arms and legs, which can form clots leading to the need for amputation. The condition is life-threatening because with a restricted flow of blood, complications arise such as pain, damage to tissue, infection and gangrene in organs and tissue, amputation, and even death. Smoking makes your blood "sticky," which is caused by the four thousand (and counting) different harmful chemicals found in cigarette smoke.

Sepsis

Out of all the causes for amputation, for me, this one hits the hardest. Sepsis almost took my life, stemming from the severe infection of my left foot. Sepsis is your body rapidly responding to severe infection; the need forbody's immune system gives up and begins fighting itself by attacking the body. The response to sepsis is life-threatening and causes organ failure tissue damage, and even death. The sepsis attack involves sending every ounce of the body's energy to the infected area, causing the body's blood-clotting mechanism to work double-time. The clots in the blood form barriers that prevent the blood from getting to major organs, causing them to fail and bring about irreparable damage to skin and tissue. What makes sepsis so severe is that your arms, legs, hands, feet, toes, and fingers are robbed of oxygen-rich blood, causing your tissue and skin to die. Sepsis moves through the body rapidly. Damage can be inflicted to all the extremities simultaneously, and when tissue and muscle are damaged beyond repair, they must be removed via amputation.

However, among the many factors and situations that cause a person to lose a limb, amputation, no matter how it happens, can be life-saving. As a new amputee, even though it can be challenging, do your best to recognize that you are alive and now it is up to you to make the best of your new life.

· 2 ·

Awaiting Amputation Surgery

Parting is inevitably painful, even for a short time. It's like an amputation, I feel a limb is being torn off, without which I shall be unable to function. And yet, once it is done . . . life rushes back into the void, richer, more vivid and fuller than before.

—Anne Morrow Lindbergh

BEFORE YOUR SURGERY

You're reading this book because you're facing amputation or have already been through the surgery. I do not know your specific situation; however, I am going to assume that you're dealing with significant infection, tissue damage, disease, or traumatic injury, and amputation has been the recommended treatment in order to save your life. Perhaps you are a family member with a loved one experiencing amputation. Either way, the goal of this book is to provide answers to significant questions about a new life as an amputee from both perspectives.

First, I want you to know you are not alone. As you face amputation, you will join the 2.1 million people in the United States known as amputees. However, losing a part of your body is a traumatic event that will significantly alter you, your body image, and your way of life. These altered images of yourself may make you feel alone, sad, and even hopeless when facing this major crisis. My intent is to help you understand that many amputees, through tenacity, perseverance, and hard work, return to a fully functioning existence. And no matter your situation, you can return to a normal life.

There are only a few cases where amputees are physically limited and not able to return to the life they once had. Mostly, these are situations where amputees have lost more than one lower limb or continue to experience ill effects of trauma, illness, or significant medical complications. The good news is that most amputees who have lost multiple limbs are able, after proper training with a prosthesis, prosthetist, or physical therapist, do return to a normal and healthy lifestyle.

Facing the reality of your new amputation will be one of the hardest aspects of your life. After limb loss the challenge is not knowing what to expect and not understanding what will happen emotionally and physically. To combat this, the first place to start a healthy and speedy recovery is through knowledge, comprehension, and understanding of what to expect.

I once visited an amputee George W. His main concern was getting back to his workplace. He was a welder by trade and had lost his left three fingers to an auto accident. His doctor had told him he probably would not be able to return to his job. His spirits were deflated because he loved his work. After some investigation, he found different companies that made specific prosthetics that could be fitted to his existing hand that would allow him to return to the job he loved. I reiterated to George that he could accomplish anything he wanted to with enough drive and determination.

UNDERSTANDING YOUR SITUATION

When I arrived at the emergency room, my left foot was inflamed, hot to the touch, and burned like fire. It was green and lifeless. Everyone around, nurses and staff, nervously looked at it and immediately called the doctor to see me. Although we were racing against the clock, my surgeon took the time to give me the facts and straight talk about anesthesia and the procedure. I admired that he took the time to explain what was happening and what could be expected after the procedure. The importance of understanding the severity of your situation is the catalyst in helping you prepare for the unknown—and for what is about to come after surgery. If your situation allows, ask about expectations before and after surgery. Ask your doctor to be open and candid about the operation and the expected results.

SURGERY PREPARATION/PLAN

Your full recovery is dependent on having a clear understanding of the entire operation and beyond. There will be some who may not want to know every detail of the procedure. Although not knowing everything can be a blessing, the severity of losing a limb makes it virtually necessary to understand what will happen following your surgery. Having a plan will prepare you and your family for the best possible recovery outcome. Make sure to ask pertinent questions before and after the procedure so you will understand what to expect with your specific situation. Having a course of action will not only help you in your recovery but assist everyone in your circles to comprehend what they will be enduring after your surgery.

QUESTIONS BEFORE SURGERY

There will be many questions you will have about your surgery and recovery and asking questions before your surgery is normal and expected. Talk to your health-care team and voice your concerns by asking questions, and remember, the only wrong question is the one not asked. To help you in learning more about your limb loss, here are some basic, pertinent questions you should ask. I left the answers generalized as your situation will differ from other amputees.

After My Surgery, When Will I Be Able to Wear a Prosthesis?

How long before you receive a prosthesis after surgery is dependent upon your age, the type and level of your amputation, your specific health condition, and the condition of your residual limb. There are multiple factors that must be addressed such as chronic illnesses, diabetes, cancer, or other diseases you may be afflicted with. Other diseases such as peripheral vascular disease, neuropathy, or peripheral artery disease can also delay healing and the fitting and wearing of your prosthesis.

If everything goes as planned and your wound heals properly, you could expect to be seen or referred to a prosthetist within approximately ninety days after your amputation. Remember, this time frame will vary from patient to patient based on how fast the wound heals from surgery. Your residual limb (stump) must have reached maximum shrinkage for proper fitting. If the prosthesis does not fit correctly, you could experience further damage to tissue around your residual limb. The fact is your body is ever-changing, and your limb will shrink over time, and the shrinkage will cause the prosthesis to loosen. This is something you will continually experience throughout your lifetime as an amputee.

Research has shown that, overall, it is easier to wear a prosthesis when the amputation is below the knee or elbow. How well you adapt to your prosthesis is purely individual and dependent upon your personal efforts overall in your recovery. Recovery from limb loss includes many variables and difficult challenges, and how you face these obstacles will determine how quickly you are ready for your prosthesis.

Many upper limb amputees prefer not to wear a prosthesis. Yet some with missing fingers choose to wear a hand prosthesis to help live more functional lives. However, most lower limb amputees depend upon their prosthesis for mobility.

How Long Will It Take for My Incision to Heal?

In most amputations, you can expect your stitches to be removed within ten to fourteen days. However, it may be necessary to leave the amputation site open because of existing infection or severe trauma. There are chronic illnesses, such as diabetes and peripheral vascular disease, that make wound healing more difficult. If you are afflicted by these kinds of diseases, make sure you have accurate information about your specific situation. Ask questions and learn about wound care and how to effectively manage your incision before leaving the hospital. This will help prevent infections for a healthy recovery.

What Will I Experience after Awakening from Surgery?

After surgery you will wake up to see your residual limb wrapped in bandages. Prepare yourself mentally for this sight because this moment will be one of the hardest of your life. It will be a shock to your system and a hard blast on your emotions. Speak to your doctor, friends, partner, or family about mentally preparing for your limb loss. Seeing your residual limb is never easy the first time, but understanding what to expect will help you cope emotionally.

Wrapping your residual limb in bandages is necessary to prevent infection and to start the important process of shrinking, which is an essential step in preparing for your new prosthesis. After surgery the pain will be intense so don't be afraid to let someone know how you are feeling. Often, many amputees are apprehensive to speak up about their pain, which could lead to experiencing further medical problems. You are the one experiencing the unique pain, so speak up and let them know where you hurt and how bad.

How Long Will I Be in the Hospital?

The duration of your hospitalization will vary and, once again, is dependent upon unique factors such as type of amputation, age, existing illnesses, or any trauma you have experienced. Hospitalization is based upon your overall physical condition before and after the surgery. There are those who heal quickly and go home right afterward. Then there are others who need rehabilitation and must spend extra time in the hospital to fully recover. Your surgeon will give you an approximate time frame. However, going home will be up to you and how your body reacts to your amputation.

How Well Will I Walk with My Amputated Leg? (Lower Limb Amputees)

This is a tough question to answer because, in the beginning, it is difficult to know how well you will adapt to your new prosthetic device. Multiple factors will include whether you have lost one leg or two and if the loss is above or below the knee. Additionally, your preexisting condition will come into play on how well you do. However, once you begin practicing with various assistive devices, you will get a general idea of how well you will walk. Practicing with devices such as canes, walkers, and crutches helps in determining your agility, physical condition, and ability to walk. Generally, people with lower level amputations adapt to walking easier. Higher, above-the-knee amputations, prove to be more challenging because of body formation and fitting issues.

Walking with your prosthesis after limb loss will be challenging, yet how soon you adapt depends on you.

How Long Will It Be before I Can Wear a Prosthesis Made for My Arm, Hand, or Fingers?

Today, prosthetic technology offers a wide range of assistive devices available for upper limb amputees. There are passive prostheses that are used for cosmetic purposes and battery-powered prostheses. There are different prostheses for arms, hands, and fingers, all designed specifically for functionality as well as aesthetics. For example, a hand prosthetic that does not move or function is merely there for cosmetic appearances. When it comes to arm and hand prosthetics, one of the most common is a prosthetic arm that is maneuvered with the body's own movements. It is designed with a special harness that fits over the torso and under the amputee's arm. There are incredible advances in upper limb prostheses where the arm or hand, and even fingers, move via battery power and small motors to ensure good grip strength.

Technological advances have produced a myoelectric prosthesis that is operated by using muscle signals from the amputee. This prosthetic device works by placing skin-surface electrodes on any existing muscles above the amputation, which then transmit a signal from the muscle movement. These devices are highly advanced, lifelike, and considered to be the greatest technology advancements in prosthetics.

Still, choosing the right device depends on your age, health, and what you foresee doing with your life. For example, if you intend to return to work or participate in your favorite sport, specific devices need to be considered. Discuss your intended lifestyle with your prosthetist to help determine the specific device best for you. The severity of your limb loss, personal preference, and health condition will also determine the particular prosthetic devices outfitted for your arm, hand, or fingers. Often, many upper limb amputees choose to not wear a prosthesis or adapt to using one sparingly. The choice is up to you.

Will I Experience Phantom Pains or Phantom Sensations?

The answer to this question is yes. In most instances you will experience phantom pains and sensations. However, they may appear immediately or later in your recovery. In *Amputation, Prosthesis Use, and Phantom*

Pain (Murray 2010), Cliff Richardson states in his chapter "Phantom Limb Pain; Prevalence, Mechanisms and Associated Factors" that a phantom pain can be described as "a continuous awareness of a (or part of a) non-existing or a deafferented body part with specific form and weight, or range of motion." Most amputees experience these sensations immediately and most describe the feelings as "pins and needles" or even "itchiness." Some phantom pains can be intense and present as actual painful feelings or (movement) called kinetic sensations. They are often described as spasms or strange moving feelings causing pain in the area. As an amputee it is normal to feel these pains because your brain is adapting to the sudden loss of your limb. Amputation, to your brain, is unexpected trauma. This immediate change to your body, even for your brain, is difficult to manage. Yet your mind goes right to work in figuring out the situation, because nerve signals are being routed to the original destination, your limb, that is no longer there. Your brain recognizes this and attempts to avert the signals elsewhere causing the pains. Remember, don't be alarmed when you experience phantom pains. They are pains and sensations that will continue throughout your amputee life.

PRESURGERY PHYSICAL CONDITION EXAMINATION

With any surgery, including amputation, you will need to undergo a thorough physical examination before the procedure takes place. Being assessed prior will help in preparing yourself for postsurgery. The medical professional conducting the examination will evaluate the strength and overall condition of the healthy remaining limbs. For example, if you are facing losing a leg, the other remaining leg should be evaluated for conditions of health and ability because it will be the primary support limb and will be taking the brunt of the workload. It must be evaluated for any outlying negative conditions. Remember, talk to your doctor if you are experiencing any problems with your body, arms, and legs.

PRESURGERY PSYCHOLOGICAL EVALUATION

Although not required in most facilities or states, an emotional or psychological evaluation should be performed before your surgery. A psychological evaluation can help with any unforeseen or underlying issues you may be experiencing. Having an understanding about your feelings prior to surgery can help you, your family, and friends cope with what is happening. A psychological assessment could show how well you will manage emotionally with the difficulty of your limb loss, which could have a dramatic impact on your psychological well-being during your recovery. A psychological evaluation could be beneficial to determine if you need additional mental support throughout your recovery.

COMING TO TERMS WITH LIMB LOSS

Limb loss either happens suddenly or is a necessary, lifesaving planned treatment. Coping with the immediate loss is necessary; at the end of the day, it always remains a personal and private affair. Whether you are surrounded by friends, a spouse, a partner, or family, you will need time for yourself to help in dealing with your loss. Reach out to your friends and family yet understand coming to terms on your own is critical to a healthy recovery.

My amputee friend Trish W. told me she wasn't ready to talk to anyone before she lost her right leg. "I needed to be with myself," she said. "I needed time alone to take it all in." Nevertheless, you may feel it necessary to speak to someone who has undergone the procedure. There are professionals and individuals among the amputee community who specialize in speaking to a new amputee. The Amputee Coalition offers the Certified Peer Visitor (CPV) Program that is designed specifically for this purpose. After my limb loss I felt compelled to give back and provide support. I became a certified peer visitor to help as many amputees as I could around the country. I've found that amputees are scared, confused, and need guidance and a helping hand. So I made it my mission to help amputees understand the severity of the situation and provide clarity, helpful guidance, and most of all to instill hope in returning to a bountiful and normal life.

Now, many amputees, and their families, contact me to talk about their limb loss, and countless others want to understand the events that take place before and after surgery. Reaching out is the first step, and vitally important, as is the essential aspect to not being afraid or ashamed to ask to talk to someone. The benefit of seeking advice and perspective from amputees who have already gone through this experience is an integral aspect to your recovery. Having an honest viewpoint can reassure you in ways never expected. Reaching out before and after your surgery is a monumental step toward a healthy and thriving recovery.

· 3 ·

Roles of Your Amputation Team

YOUR AMPUTATION AND YOUR TEAM

Surgery and recovery will involve multiple members of a health-care team. Each member will perform essential functions to aid in a full recovery. Limb loss recovery has specific treatment methods where working closely with many individuals is essential. During these treatments strong bonds and relationships develop, which provide necessary support, encouragement, and peace of mind knowing that people are behind you and want to see you succeed. Ralph Waldo Emerson wrote, "To know even one life has breathed easier because you have lived. This is to have succeeded." Remember, everyone on your team wants to inspire, guide, and motivate you along each step of your recovery. Still, the healthy path toward a strong recovery includes fully understanding the specific roles each member of your amputation team performs. Perhaps you are a family member experiencing amputation alongside a loved one, the members of the health-care team will have a significant impact on your life as well.

Learning the role of each team member helps everyone to make the best decisions for your care. Every member of your health-care team should provide insight and guidance through the critical time before and after surgery. Different members of your team may include:

- General surgeon
- Primary care physician
- Nurses
- Physical therapist

- Occupational therapist
- Rehabilitation specialist
- Prosthetist
- Podiatrist
- Social worker
- Psychologist

Your Surgeon

Amputation surgeons have a unique role and responsibility in your limb loss journey. Most surgeons strive for a safe removal of the damaged or diseased limb while simultaneously working on reconstructing your remaining limb. The restoration is essential to prepare for your prosthesis along with proper wound healing. Skilled amputation surgeons understand the importance and long-term effects of proper amputation surgical technique on a patient's postsurgery outcome. The amputation surgeon must know not only the amputation procedure itself, but also possess the understanding of rehabilitation, healing, and limb loss physiology. To accomplish this most surgeons utilize a team approach and take advantage of the skills and know-how of his trusted team to provide you with the best care.

Your Primary Care Physician

Your general physician or primary care doctor is your go-to team member for all your medical needs. A general practitioner will play an integral role in your recovery and further health after your amputation. There will be many professionals surrounding you while in recovery, yet the one vital person is your primary doctor. Remember to continue to see your family doctor to ensure that you remain on the right track with your recovery. Your health and successful recovery depend on the primary doctor to be the go-to defense mechanism in maintaining excellent health and preventive care with your limb loss.

Nurses

I cannot speak higher praises for these skilled professionals who work the front lines of health care. Nurses are essential to taking care of your medical needs before and after surgery. These talented people are trained professionals who provide up-close personal care and administer necessary medications and wound treatment. Many nurses, because of their close-knit ties to their patients, could become a confidant and cheerleader throughout your recovery.

Physical Therapist

Physical therapists play a vital role in your limb loss recovery, which will include working one-on-one with your physical therapist to prepare for the fitting and wearing of your prosthesis. The prosthesis plan begins immediately after surgery with physical therapists who are trained to aid in mobility issues, strength training, balance, and using assistive devices to keep you mobile. The essential goal of a physical therapist is to provide the best direction toward returning to a normal life. Physical therapy is vital to your new physical as well as emotional life. Without physical therapy, many unforeseen problems during and after your recovery could emerge. Even after your recovery, a physical therapist may be necessary because through daily use, your prosthesis's condition, or problems healthwise, might wane, causing balance and mobility problems.

Remember, physical therapy is vital, yet will be an immense challenge, so do your best, work hard, listen, and step up to the challenge.

Occupational Therapist

Occupational therapy is an often overlooked, yet essential aspect of your recovery. Working with an occupational therapist provides support, guidance, and superior motivation toward managing and coping with daily activities to get you back to living a normal life. Most occupational therapists deliver specific one-on-one rehabilitation and prosthetic training.

An occupational therapist provides many essential services, such as:

- Examining your functional goals. They help you with your self-care, work-related tasks, home, and workplace management. Plus, they assist you with mobility, driving, personal activities, family, and childcare.

- Evaluating your daily routine and help with suggested modifications to accomplish tasks.
- Employing educational information on specific amputation techniques and teach about prosthetic accessories and how to use them to accomplish daily tasks and return to normal living.
- Helping you with your prosthetic training.
- Addressing any emotional issues you are experiencing.

Rehabilitation Specialist

Throughout the past few decades, rehabilitation specialists and professional growth and development workers have emerged as essential caregivers to the amputee community. Rehabilitation specialists manage vocational and disability issues and work with disabled veteran programs, state-to-state disability programs, along with federal and state workers' compensation programs. Many of today's rehabilitation specialists work in a broad range of cases generating exceptional results and personal rewards. After limb loss your recovery could involve working with a rehabilitation therapist. These skilled professionals specialize in rehabilitation of amputations such as upper limb, hand, arms, and lower limb. Many rehabilitation specialists are certified and licensed in psychosocial and medical treatments and can help amputees with mental issues and emotional trauma, along with the physical aspect of injuries. The goal of working with a rehabilitation specialist is to help you be fully functional in your daily life and activities. Ask your healthcare team about meeting a rehabilitation specialist that fits best with your specific limb loss.

Prosthetist

A prosthetist is a critical element and vital member of your health-care team and prosthetic life. A prosthetist will work with you one-on-one in the fitting and making of your new prosthesis. Choosing a prosthetist is important because you will meet with them often for extended periods, and because of the nature of the prosthetist/patient relationship, bonds are formed through close-knit discussions. Cynthia W., one of my close amputee friends, told me she adored her prosthetist. "We got really close," she said. "She and I formed a special bond from the visits and how well she helped me through it all."

While working with your prosthetist, being transparent about your needs and goals is critical to a positive recovery outcome. Go over what you want to accomplish and explain your vision of your life. Whether it's getting back to work, recreation, or level of activity, let them know because life plans coincide with a proper fitting and design of your prosthesis. Understanding your plans aids the prosthetist in the design of a specific prosthesis that will meet your goals and expectations.

Once your prosthesis is designed and fitted, let your prosthetist know precisely how it feels and fits. Any prosthesis must be comfortable, not cause pain, or be uncomfortable. A poor fit that causes pain can hinder your desire to use it, which can prevent you from pursuing activities that you want. A good fit is critical so that pressure points don't cause severe irritation, chaffing, pain, skin breakdown, and calluses, which can lead to open wounds, infections, and possible disastrous problems.

Podiatrist

One of the major problems with amputations of a lower limb is proper care of the healthy remaining limb. Many amputees have complications such as diabetes and neuropathy that require close-knit care. If you have diabetes and have now experienced a lower limb amputation because of the complications of the disease, proper foot care is essential to avoid further problems compromising your healthy foot. Foot ulcers and wounds are the number one complication stemming from diabetes and neuropathy because neuropathy causes numbness and no natural sign or detection of pain. This complication leads to injuries being undetected and becoming infected, steering you to significant trouble and possibly placing you at risk of losing the healthy limb.

However, many people with diabetes can diminish their risk and prevent amputation of their sound limbs with proper diabetic management, immediate wound care, and regular foot exams by a trained and certified podiatrist. Practicing daily foot care is essential by checking your feet twice a day. Look for swelling, redness, small cuts, or blisters. As a diabetic amputee, never trim your own toenails. This task of cutting and trimming your toenails must be left up to a professional podiatrist. Cutting the toenails too short can cause minor cuts and abrasions that can lead to infection. The rule to live by is to avoid "bathroom surgery" and schedule regular visits to your podiatrist who has the proper equipment and tools to treat your feet and toenails safely.

Social Worker

Social workers provide mental and emotional support during this transitional time. A social worker provides you relief from the cumbersome tasks to allow a smooth transition home. These highly trained workers help with tasks such as locating insurance carriers, home health care, and scheduling of assistive devices needed for mobility within your home. Returning home is a joyous yet fearful time, and, through the help of a social worker, is the beginning of adapting to your new situation. I recently spoke to a right-leg below-the-knee amputee, James P., who was apprehensive about going home. I told him that going home was the first step in figuring things out on his own. James said, "I'm scared to be alone and on my own with a missing leg. Honestly, I'm scared to death." So I arranged a meeting with James's social worker to go over some logistics to make him feel better about the home transition. He was able to go home more secure, with no problems.

Social workers provide insightful information for you and your family to begin your new limb loss journey. Remember, limb loss requires many things, not just mobility but coordination of your mind, body, and spirit. And this is where social workers use their expertise by providing resources for patients to help with the challenges of returning home and dealing with the complications of amputee life. Social workers assist in transitional care and focus on what is needed to return home effectively. The good news is that most social workers also assist everyone in your circle affected by your limb loss. The goal is to help everyone cope with the situation from different perspectives—children, spouses, parents, and siblings.

Psychologist

Human nature is most vulnerable when losing a limb because of the multitude of associated emotions that emerge. These emotions can appear early on or years later, so speaking to a professional psychiatrist can help sort through the deep-rooted emotions you may be experiencing. Emotional outbursts could happen when you least expect them and can escalate to dangerous levels and become out of your control. A psychologist plays an integral role with your emotional well-being with a limb loss. Do not take your emotions lightly because even though they may not appear severe, they could wreak havoc in your life.

When you feel out of sorts or your emotions feel out of control, speak to a psychologist as soon as possible. Remember, a psychologist is trained to assist with helping you cope. With everything you're feeling, do your best to remain open about your feelings and what you are experiencing. Speaking with someone who understands is a humbling step, yet monumental in the recovery process. I have experienced an array of mixed emotions and have come to embrace talking with my therapist. There isn't any shame in doing so. Charles Dickens, in *Great Expectations*, wrote, "We need never be ashamed of our tears." Limb loss is filled with heavy tears, cumbersome effort, and burdensome emotions at various levels, and often we merely need help. Utilize the knowledge received from your psychologist because it could prove useful, even lifesaving, during your recovery.

Every amputee has a health-care recovery team. It is vital to understand the roles each member plays within your recovery and use their specific skills to help you reach a healthy outcome. Amputation is life-changing and filled with obstacles, difficulties, and challenges, yet you will endure through the help of others. You will make it because your health-care recovery team will work stringently by implementing their expertise to ensure you the best recovery possible. Remember, Rome wasn't built in a day, and it will take time, effort, tenacity, pure heart, and fortitude to get yourself back to living a normal life. Limb loss takes an immense amount of guts and belief in yourself along with the help of others to do what it is necessary in getting your life back.

III

AFTER THE AMPUTATION: PHYSICAL RECOVERY

After Amputation Surgery

What to Expect

> My advice to other disabled people would be, concentrate
> on things your disability doesn't prevent you doing well,
> and don't regret the things it interferes with. Don't be
> disabled in spirit as well as physically.
>
> —Stephen Hawking

*J*ennifer M. woke up in the hospital and said, "All I can remember is the crashing of the metal as the van turned over and over. Everything was spinning, and I felt a powerful pull on my left arm. I didn't feel any pain at first, but as the van stopped, I could see my arm was torn off. It was gone, above the elbow."

Accidents, such as this, happen every day, and whether or not expected, you are now officially an amputee. Gracie Rosenberg (2018), a double lower amputee and founder of Standing with Hope, an organization that provides prosthetic limbs for those in need, said in her article "Living with Amputation: Gracie Rosenberger's Story,"

> I have endured 71 operations and still live with extreme pain, but I
> now know there is life on the other side of amputation. Some things
> in our lives can become so badly damaged that it literally cripples us
> to keep them. In my case, letting go of my legs allowed me to get
> where I am today, living an active life full of meaning and purpose.
> Just because you're missing some parts doesn't change who you are.
> In fact, it may bring out who you truly are. ·

An immense adjustment is necessary after limb loss, the largest being coming to terms with your loss. Seeing the amputation site for the first time will bring on intense physical and emotional pains. This emotional roller-coaster can be devastating and difficult to understand initially. When I first saw my amputation and the massive amount of dressings and bandages surrounding my leg, my heart shattered. I hung my head and cried. I felt helpless, writhing in pain, heartbroken, and facing a life I never imagined for myself. That first glimpse was a moment frozen in time, etched deeply into my memory. It hurt to see the sheet lying flat, motionless, where my left leg should have been. Everything in my world stopped; I was the image of an altered man, broken, confused, and, most of all, unsure of the future. In those first seconds my mind burned with questions. I wondered how I was ever going to come back from this; it shattered my world into a million pieces, and I didn't see how I ever could. What was unbelievable to me was that my left leg, below the knee, was undeniably gone forever.

How an amputee manages themselves after limb loss has been thoroughly explored, yet not fully understood because everyone reacts to circumstances differently. The initial sight of your missing limb can affect you in ways you never expect or comprehend. Losing a limb is intense, emotional, and painful in more ways than physical because limb loss is unnerving and may cause intense shock, and you may react by disconnecting from the situation. Removing ourselves from things that hurt is a human instinct. Withdrawal is a natural way to avoid emotional and physical pain. Experiencing deep, confusing emotions is a normal reaction after limb loss. "I didn't know how to feel," Jim W. told me during a Certified Peer Visit visit. He continued, "I was stunned and didn't want to see my right leg gone. But I knew I had to, eventually."

No one can deny the harshness of the initial sight and the inner turmoil that follows. Still, only you know what and how you feel. Remember, this is your time to endure the wave of feelings as they come. Many amputees I have spoken with report experiencing a cascade of initial emotions such as anger, anxiety, confusion, and frustration. Some of those feelings are either directed inward toward themselves or outward toward family members. Later, deeper feelings of depression, denial, hopelessness, numbness, and even helplessness can appear.

Dee Malchow, the author of *Alive & Whole: Amputation: Emotional Recovery* (2016), describes her feelings after her amputation surgery:

> This time, as I revived momentarily in the recovery room, I raised
> my head and glanced briefly at my right lower extremity. No foot

or leg lifted the sheet in the natural form that had been there for 19 years. It was flat . . . empty. I rested my head back on the pillow with great sadness, but also an odd sense of relief. It's over, and I breathed silently. But it had only begun.

Obviously, Dee felt a sense of relief as some amputees do after surgery. They feel lifted from the burden of pain, discomfort, and worry suffered from wounds and other health issues. Everyone is different and will experience varying levels of emotions after limb loss. Emotions are a deep personal experience, and coping requires dealing with each emotion the best way you can. When you feel out of control or lost, talk with a professional. Confide in a family member or your doctor about what you are feeling, because emotions could feel like a roller-coaster with extreme highs and deep lows. During your recovery emotions could make you feel out of control or strange inside. One minute you could feel positive and optimistic and the next filled with despair. Pay close attention to yourself and how you feel. Do your best to not let things get out of control.

Over time unmanaged emotions can drastically affect your life. Everything from your attention, concentration, and ability to focus can be compromised. During a peer visit, Sarah P., a right leg amputee, said to me, "I felt out of control and as if I was going out of my mind." "Don't worry," I said, "Being aware of how you feel is the first positive step." Remember, everything you endure now, with time, will ease. The key is to be aware of what you are experiencing. However, if it deeply troubles you, do not hesitate in seeking professional help or speaking to your doctor. Physical and emotional healing starts immediately after surgery, and coming to terms with your loss is an integral part of a successful recovery. Amputation is a massive loss, comparable to death, and the first step in recovery is allowing yourself the freedom and time to grieve. It is vital to let it out. This is your personal time to feel sorrow.

PHYSICAL PAIN—THE FIRST HOURS

When my amputee friend Scott W. was coming out of anesthesia, he felt a sharp pain shooting through his left leg. The pain went all the way into what seemed were his missing toes. "I was groggy and not entirely coherent," Scott said, "but the strange feelings I felt were so strong that I believed that my toes and leg were still there. I cried. And for a split second, I was oddly relieved from the sensations. They felt like the amputation never happened and my leg and foot were still there." At first Scott thought a miracle happened, and the surgeon had saved his leg and foot. However, this wasn't the case. The feelings Scott experienced are called Phantom Limb Syndrome, which involves the nerves and brain reacting to the sudden removal of the limb. My limb loss included immediate sensations of my missing toes moving and everything with my senses were scrambled from the genuine pain of my missing limb. The hardest thing to grasp was the reality of seeing my missing foot, yet the sensations coming from the amputation sight were distinct and strangely real. Still, there wasn't anything I could do—I could not escape.

Pain. We have all experienced it. From falling off your first bicycle to stubbing your toe, pain comes in various degrees. However, everyone's pain threshold is different. The intense discomfort you experience after amputation is a tangled web of feelings, nerves, and emotions. What escalates the situation are the strange biting sensations that accompany the deep emotions. Pain around your residual limb will be intense, yet some will be phantom sensations. Some amputees say they don't have these feelings at first but end up experiencing them later. Scientists believe phantom sensations are your body and brain doing its best to route the nerve signals to the correct destination. Phantom sensations originate in your spinal cord and are signals from your brain and the nerves associated with the missing limb. The brain goes to work and continues emitting nerve signals as the body desperately tries to figure out where to send them. This causes a massive tangle of nerve signals, which cross paths, creating shooting pains and sensations at the location of the amputation.

Whether through a traumatic accident or planned surgery, for the brain, amputation is abrupt, and the body has built-in triggers sensing when things are wrong. This is our reptilian brain taking action, starting with the fight-or-flight response to the nervous system. Fight-or-flight is the body's natural response to any perceived threat or danger. Hormones such as adrenalin and cortisol are released, increasing the rate of the heart and altering multiple autonomic nervous functions, allowing the body to react with strength and energy. The term "fight-or-flight" comes from the body's ability to fight or flee when faced with danger or pain. When the body believes the threat is gone, it reverts to a normal state. However, in most stressful events such as limb loss, returning to a normal state is delayed, causing further damage to the body.

With amputation your body goes into alarm mode telling the brain something is wrong and converts those signals into intense pain. Although the immediate pain is normal, some studies have discovered that your brain and body will continuously work to correct it. The brain will try to return to a normal state by remapping the sensory nerves and sending the signals to other parts of your body. For example, the nerves going to your missing limb could be sent to your forehead, arm, or any other healthy body part that shouldn't experience pain.

BUILDING STRENGTH

Getting an amputee patient active as soon as possible is a stance many doctors adopt after surgery. My good friend, Thomas M., a right-leg below-the-knee amputee, had a unique experience of getting active early in his recovery. He said,

> I set a goal to transition from the bed to a chair as soon as possible. I had been in the hospital bed and I craved sitting upright in a comfortable chair. So, I swung my legs out and the momentum of my body weight pulled me straight to the hospital floor. I landed directly on the bone of my amputated limb, and it hurt like hell. The nurses came running, but instead of picking me up, the nurse said, "You need to do this yourself." The pain was intense, but I was able to get myself up and into the chair.

That moment was an eye-opener for Thomas because he learned how quickly mishaps occur, and yet, through his fall, there was a breakthrough and, most of all, discovery of himself. Thomas found in that moment he could accomplish remarkable things—on his own.

Once I started getting physical therapy and using a walker, I embraced the challenge. In the beginning, I took small steps. As I took more steps, my confidence grew. Before long I was adding more, pushing myself, gaining more strength and confidence. Those incremental steps were giant leaps in my recovery because I was able to adapt, overcome, and discover ways to gain freedom and comfort. The pain, sweat, and tears I endured taught me more about myself and showed me that my true capabilities were endless. Everything was up to me.

With physical therapy and devices, listen, work hard, and push yourself through your physical therapy and recovery. Author Daniel H. Wilson said, "The goal for many amputees is no longer to reach a 'natural' level of ability but to exceed it, using whatever cutting-edge technology is available. As this new generation sees it, our tools are evolving faster than the human body, so why obey the limits of mere nature?" Leah Labelle, *American Idol* contestant said, "Work hard for what you want because it won't come to you without a fight. You have to be strong and courageous and know that you can do anything you put your mind to."

Building strength will be an immense challenge, and in this moment your goal is to endure the pain, fight through it, and strive to make yourself strong. Will it be easy? No, it will not. Over the next few weeks your body and mind will fight you. Remember, the body wants to be in a comfortable state, and yet, over time, it will readjust the sensory information it has known your entire life. So, each day rise up, work hard, and soon you'll notice the pain will lessen, making everything more tolerable. Once the pain is manageable, you will engage in more activity, which aids in gaining confidence and feeling better about yourself. Being mobile will bring you one step closer to living the new life that is yours to live.

HOW LONG WILL MY RECOVERY BE?

Rudolf Breuss, an Austrian scientist and author of *The Breuss Cancer Cure* (1995), said, "To my mind, healing means returning a malfunctioning human body to full unrestricted function, not to remove parts of it by operation or amputation." How long your recovery takes depends upon any preexisting health conditions and your specific limb loss, whether upper or lower. However, hospitalization will be longer if you are a lower extremity amputee, because on average you could expect to leave the hospital in about two to three weeks. Recovery after lower limb amputation is a delicate dance because the complications can be complex and lead to longer hospital stays. Lower extremity recovery involves learning how to walk again, weight-bearing training with physical therapy, and rehabilitation sessions. A lower extremity amputee's recovery involves strengthening groups of different muscles while learning to safely transfer between various areas and obstacles such as from bed to chair or wheelchair. Expect to practice and develop mobility by using several walking devices such as crutches, walkers, and wheelchairs. These assistive devices are designed to help you build stamina, provide mobility, and learn daily living skills. Mobility and strengthening will help you with confidence and be independent before returning home.

If you are an upper extremity amputee, you can expect less time in the hospital. The stay could average between three to seven days, and because of the shorter recovery time, many upper limb amputees begin preparation for a prosthesis in a short amount of time. As with any amputee, you, as an upper extremity amputee, must first recognize and start trying to cope with what has changed in your life. Upper extremity amputees must address how to overcome and adapt to the use of a prosthesis or go without one to manage tasks within your daily life. Managing your limb loss will include working with physiotherapists who will help strengthen various muscles to prepare for your prosthesis. There is a lot to learn, and all is essential in order for the new prosthesis to function with once routine daily tasks. Effective rehabilitation methods involve adapting to new skills that improve upper extremity functionality. Expect to work with not only physiotherapists but also occupational therapists using strengthening exercises, virtual reality, and different mirror therapies. Remember, stay with it. Learning to maneuver your prosthetic will take time, effort, and persistence. All you do will increase your independence, which is a critical aspect of getting your life back in order.

There are many new and remarkable prosthetic technologies for upper extremity amputees that have been developed along with strong advancements in prosthetic designs. These vast improvements in prosthetic design have helped many patients return to a normal life in a shorter amount of time. With these new prosthetic artificial limbs, patients achieve feats never seen in the early stages of limb loss, gripping objects, handling tools, writing, or even playing guitar.

Remember, through it all, depending on your condition of health and complications, recovery could take longer. Be patient. If you face an extended stay in the hospital, talk to your family and become prepared for the additional time by bringing fresh clothes, supplies, and money in case you need to get haircuts or buy anything ancillary while you are there. While there, take the extra time to work hard, prepare, and push yourself through the physical therapy to get out and on your way to a healthy recovery.

Major Complications after Amputation

$\mathcal{A}$ month and half after losing my left leg, the large incision site was almost healed. However, one evening, still in a wheelchair, I saw a large wet spot on the bandage surrounding my incision. My wife and I removed the bandage to find a small part of the incision oozing. Frantic, she and I drove straight to the emergency room. "I do not see any infection," the doctor said. "Looks like some typical drainage around the incision site. Go home and keep an eye on it, and if anything feels or gets worse, come back immediately." I was in doubt of the medical prognosis because I was petrified of getting another infection and losing more of my leg. However, my wife and I went home as instructed. The next day I felt fine and examined the incision site. It looked good. Nonetheless, within three hours, I had a raging fever with massive blobs of infection dripping from my leg. We sped back to the emergency room, and the doctors and nurses frantically treated the infection to prevent it from getting worse. The doctors gave me a shot of a powerful antibiotic, Rocephin. My heart pounded as I faced the harsh reality that I was extremely vulnerable to germs, bacteria, and infection, and probably will be the rest of my life. This event showed me that I needed to be vigilant with self-monitoring to remain safe and healthy to alleviate further complications.

Setbacks after amputation are a significant concern because challenging difficulties can arise throughout your recovery that you need to be aware of. Remember, only you can continuously monitor your condition and inform people around you what you are experiencing. There is an undeniable responsibility to yourself because only you can tell someone how you are hurting. The pain and discomfort from complications could be intense and should not be ignored. Major complications need immediate attention before irreparable damage occurs.

To help in recognizing complications, let's look at a few problematic issues you could experience.

WOUNDS AND INFECTIONS

Wounds and infections are common complications after limb loss surgery, and if you are a diabetic, you could endure slower healing of your incision. Research has shown that of all nontraumatic amputations in the United States, 60 percent are performed on people with diabetes. Throughout the world it's estimated that every thirty seconds an amputation takes place because of diabetes. Many diabetics experience neuropathic pain known as neuropathy, which make injuries, wounds, and sores undetectable due to metabolic changes in the peripheral and central nervous systems. Peripheral neuropathy is numbness of the nerves that prevent pain receptors from detecting or alerting the brain of pain from injuries or wounds. Not being able to feel pain is one of the major causes severe complications including amputation. These factors make it necessary to check your body vigilantly.

Diabetes is not the only cause of wounds and complications after surgery. Other injuries and infections of the surgical site after amputation are a significant concern. Surgical site infection is common and has adverse effects on healing and recovery time. Complications from wounds and infection can affect levels of phantom pain, and even alter the eventual fitting of the prosthetic. A 2014 study of Medicare data showed that chronic, nonhealing wounds and associated complications affect nearly 15 percent or 8.2 million Medicare beneficiaries. Most of the wounds were found to be associated with infected or reopened surgical sites. Early identification of any complication from wounds or potential infections can mean the difference in having a positive outcome or not.

BURSAE BONE

Adventitious bursae are a major complication that occurs, mostly after lower extremity amputation. This complication happens when friction, pressure, and the continual motion of skin over the bone takes place causing intense pain. To avoid this problem, if you're a lower extremity amputee, your doctor can prescribe a unique sock called a stump-shrinker sock, which is designed to provide constant pressure on your residual leg, speeding up the shrinking and movement of tissue and preventing the formation of bursae bone. Additionally, the stump-shrinking sock allows for the best fit of your prosthetic. Bursae bone creates painful complications because as the bone significantly grows, it causes immense pain and discomfort inside and outside the prosthetic. Further, the enlargement of the bone can cause a prosthetic not to fit correctly. An improper fit could cause pain and deter you from wearing your prosthetic.

EDEMA

Edema is an excessive accumulation of fluid in the tissue and cavities of the body. Amputation is trauma and injury to your body, and edema is a natural inflammatory response to your injury with excessive fluid causing swelling around the wound. As you heal, the fluid and swelling dissipates, reducing the size of the stump. Your doctor may employ different methods to quickly minimize the edema before starting the process of prosthetic fitting. Decreasing the size of your stump is essential in beginning the phase of prosthetic preparation. For a proper initial fit, the residual limb must be the appropriate size for adequate measurement, fitting, and shaping of your prosthetic socket.

MUSCLE WEAKNESS

During the beginning stages of your recovery, muscle weakness in your healthy limb is to be expected. The sooner physical therapy is introduced, the better your recovery. For lower limb amputees, muscle weakness after amputation causes problems of instability and balance issues. Strengthening the healthy limbs or digits is critical, along with increasing strength and power throughout the entire body. Strength training of your remaining limb will stave off pain, stiffness, and spasms, which cause significant discomfort in the joints and muscles.

When a limb is amputated, the remaining muscle mass could be lost and cause reduced strength and decreased mobility. As a lower amputee, in the first few days and weeks you are mostly bedridden. When in this state it becomes incredibly challenging to remain mobile. Being immobile for longer durations causes intense muscle weakness. If you are an upper extremity amputee you may not be bedridden, yet there still can be apparent issues of muscle weakness in your joints and remaining extremities. Physical therapy and rehabilitation will assist in relieving muscle weakness by including exercise programs, gait training, and assist device mobility sessions, all tailored for strengthening muscles and building stamina.

CONTRACTURES

Becoming as mobile and active as you can early on helps avoid contractures, which are the shortening of joints due to tightness in the tendons, skin, and muscles as a result of inactivity. One symptom of contracture is when your skin loses its elasticity and becomes unable to stretch, limiting your movements. Contractures are seen after traumatic events such as amputation, burns, and prolonged limitation of the movement of a limb. The initial inactivity associated with lower extremity amputees can lead to contractures, so close attention to any painful area on your limb, inflammation, and restricted movement. If you experience these symptoms, please tell your caregiver or doctor right way.

OPENING OF A WOUND OR INCISION

Two days after my friend Marie D.'s amputation she almost hurt herself badly. She had to use the bathroom, and as she swung her right leg out of bed, she completely forgot that she didn't have a left leg any longer. Her mind hadn't yet registered the trauma to her body. Her weight and momentum pulled her out of bed and onto the floor. She crashed, landing straight down on the bone of her leg.

"I felt the jolt into my teeth," she said.

Marie's leg had been amputated guillotine-style, and the bone, muscle, and tissue were exposed—even though wrapped in bandages, it was open and was not sutured up. So, when she hit the floor, it was a direct hit onto her bone but did not damage or tear away any of the remaining tissue.

"I thought I had done a number on myself," she said. "But, fortunately, I did not damage anything, and it was a close call."

As a lower limb amputee, during the first days and weeks of recovery, there is risk of falling or tearing of the incision once you start to be mobile. Being human and prone to accidents, falls or tripping over miscellaneous items is now a major concern. If you are a lower limb amputee, loss of balance is an important factor to consider as it increases the risk of falling so accidents with mobility devices happen often because of lack of strength and balance problems, causing sudden falls. A fall can be a significant complication, causing exposure of bone and muscle. So you must take all precautions to protect yourself from any direct fall or trauma.

TISSUE NECROSIS

Necrosis or tissue necrosis is described as the unnatural death of cells and tissue caused by physical injury, lack of oxygen or blood flow, and infections. Tissue necrosis happens when tissue dies near and around your surgery site. Diabetic amputees are at greater risk of tissue necrosis due to possible lack of blood flow to the stump area from existing vascular disease or neuropathy. Tissues necrosis can be identified by seeing dark changes in areas of your skin. If you have ever witnessed a homeless person with black feet, this is a sign of tissue necrosis. With tissue necrosis, your skin and tissue break down, which leads to further complications and risk of infection. Tissue necrosis could be severe and cause further damage to your body and even lead to death. Throughout your recovery examine your body and stump area daily. If you see any discoloration, puffiness, swelling, or anything out of the ordinary, please seek your doctor or emergency help.

SKIN BLISTERS

Skin blisters are a complication caused by bandage dressings around your incision. As an amputee, blisters are something you will need to be aware of the rest of your days. The tension from bandages or a prosthesis reduces movement and the breathing of the skin, causing blisters to form. Blisters can also be formed from an allergic reaction to the adhesive on bandages and dressings. Pay close attention to your body at every stage, examine yourself thoroughly, and take matters into your own hands. Remember, it is up to you to keep up on your personal conditions and well-being.

NOCICEPTIVE PAINS IN THE STUMP

When it comes to pain after amputation, one-third of amputees have some form of nociceptive pain. This kind of pain is apparent for various reasons and can be linked to issues such as:

- Localized wound infection pain
- Abnormal stump issues post-op
- Allergic reactions to bandages, tape, gauze
- Allergic reactions to prosthetic accessories (stump liners, stump socks, prosthesis materials)
- Skin and incision pain
- Tissue and muscle pain from ill-fitting prosthesis sockets

After coming out of surgery, I felt cramping as if my foot and toes were still there. However, I saw massive bandages around my left leg. Once fully awake, I was in total sensory overload. Jolts of pain burned like hot coals in my residual leg.

Most amputees report the nociceptive pain weeks and months after surgery with weird sensations, blasts of pain that feel like stabbing, burning, throbbing, shooting, and even cramping that come without warning. To a new amputee these feelings can be unnerving, confusing, and considered a major complication.

When you experience this kind of pain, talk with your doctor or health-care provider immediately. Pain like this is part of your journey to recovery, and yet it can be frightening. However, even though extreme and unpleasant, you can beat it.

TAKING CARE OF YOURSELF AND YOUR HEALTH

One of the essential aspects of an optimal recovery after limb loss is taking care of your health and following advice on all treatment plans. Stringently monitoring your overall health will play a significant role in getting your incision to heal properly. After surgery your incision is vulnerable to problematic aspects such as germs, bacteria and allergic reactions. These issues can cause wounds and irritation and grow into full-blown infections. Mike W., one of my close amputee friends, told me, "I noticed redness around the top of my stump. At first, I just thought it was irritated, but I was wrong. The redness got worse and I saw infection pouring out, so my wife rushed me to the emergency room. They got it in time, and I'm so glad they did because the doctors told me it was about to turn into something worse. I could have lost more of my leg."

Train yourself to spot problems and abnormal issues with your stump and body. Pay close attention every day for any problems by inspecting yourself from head to toe. Take time to examine the harder areas such as your back, between your toes, end of your stump, or the bottom of your feet. Have a trusted family member inspect unreachable areas at least twice a week. Examining your body will save you pain and grief down the road. If you spot a wound or an issue anywhere on your body, see your doctor right away.

Amputation life is surrounded with a varying degree of complications, and the first step is to understand your body, listen, and pay close attention throughout your recovery. If you experience any of these complications it is critical to speak with your doctor or seek emergency care. Remember, humans make mistakes, and sometimes, even under the best care, complications still arise and could go undiscovered. No one can feel what you are experiencing. You are the only one. Even with immense support and medical care, at the end of the day, your entire recovery is up to you. Empower yourself by making your health, body, and mind top priority to get back to a healthy and normal life.

· 6 ·

Going Home

A New Life Journey

INGRESS AND EGRESS:
GETTING IN AND OUT OF YOUR HOME

$\mathcal{G}$etting out of the hospital and going home is a monumental step in your overall recovery. Leaving the hospital is an exciting moment and provides you a newfound freedom, a positive step forward in your limb loss journey. Yet if you are a lower limb amputee, going home could be challenging and even problematic. With lower limb loss and the nature of mobility with getting in and out of the home, strategic planning is needed for this transition. The goal is to return home comfortably, easily, and safely. Once, during a certified peer visit, I met Terry W., a right-leg below-the-knee amputee. She was scheduled to be released to go home in a few short days. So I asked her, "What are your plans, and how do you feel about going home?" She responded, "Well, I hope my daily life gets back to normal. But look at me, is there such a thing as normal anymore?" I admit her statement took me aback. I remained silent, but before I could answer, she said, "I'm sure I will need to learn to do things differently than others at home. I guess it is all a part of learning what I can do and can't do. The only thing I must do is not let my limb loss hinder my ability to try."

She was right.

Understanding that things will be different will involve patience, ingenuity, and acceptance for the best outcome is important when transitioning to home. The best approach to adapting in returning to your home is planning and taking it one day at a time. Another left-leg amputee friend, Audrey B., said, "I am most afraid of stairs when I get home. I'm not sure if I can go up and down safely. Plus, I'm afraid of being too slow around my family." I told her to approach climbing the stairs just like everything else in her life—one step at a time. I advised her to not worry about being slow. Family should be understanding and accommodating to your condition. Returning home involves keeping realistic expectations and taking charge of your daily life. Embrace what your new life has to offer, understand your limits, and recognize your immense capabilities. Living at home is the beginning of it all.

Having a strategic plan is essential for you and your love ones when going home. This will make the return home easier for everyone. If you are a lower limb amputee, going in and out (ingress and egress) is an essential factor to consider, so plan accordingly for your comfort and safety. Some houses are older and designed for people without disabilities, so going in and out may be problematic. Initially, before returning home, have a professional occupational therapist or rehabilitation specialist evaluate the layout and design of your home to develop a proper and safe plan of return. On the exterior of your home, have the following looked at closely:

- Stairs to the front door
- Stairs to the back door
- Walkways: front and back
- Sidewalks: front and back
- Driveway: ingress through the garage

Coordinate and discuss a plan to maneuver in, out, and around your home with your family and caregivers. Take the time and draw a mock property and floor plan to evaluate the best approach. As a lower limb amputee, evaluating the floor plan is important when a wheelchair or other assistive devices will be used in the home. "I had to make sure I could get through the house," Tina S., a double-leg above-the-knee amputee, told me during a CPV visit. "I had my husband move the furniture around so I could wheel around easier." This is good advice. Ask your family to help you prepare your home's interior by moving furniture and limiting obstacles to help you safely get around. Look for items such as:

- Electrical cords
- Loose floor rugs

- Interior steps
- Stairways
- Entryways
- Door facings (width for wheelchairs)
- Odds and ends
- Miscellaneous furniture

If you need assistance in planning to go home, talk to a social worker or occupational therapist on getting help. My good friend Sam T., a right-leg above-the-knee amputee, said, "I sat down and drew the layout of my house while in the hospital. I had time and I knew I needed to come up with a plan to help my wife and family help me get around." Consider your home's design; examine stairs and porches that provide access to the front and rear doors. Are there stairs to the front door? Are there stair rails outside to help you? Can you access the front door easily? If not, you may need a wheelchair ramp, which could be a major cost to consider.

After my limb loss, my wife and I sat down and quickly discovered that a wheelchair ramp was needed on the side door of our home to allow me to get in and out. With some help from friends, we had a ramp built before I returned home. Knowing it was there helped me feel more secure and confident and transition easier.

If you discover the need for a wheelchair ramp, and if finances are an issue, there are organizations that can help secure funds for tasks such as building an accessible ramp or for assist devices. The U.S. Department of Veterans Affairs offers two different grants: the Specially Adapted Housing Grant and the Special Housing Adaptation Grant. The Think Alive Foundation in Amherst, Massachusetts, partners with the Special Education Parent Advisory Council to offer a limited number of grants designed for youths twenty-one and under. The grants can be used for minor home modifications costing from $50 to $500 to help a child with a disability in making a safer environment in and around the house. Rebuilding Together Americorps members build new homes or modify existing ones for people living with a disability. The Rural Housing Repair Loans and Grants program, which is funded by the USDA, provides funds to be used to modify existing residences or to install new home features making living quarters safer. In order to qualify, you must be sixty-two years old or more and from a low-income household. The American Red Cross provides financial assistance to military service members. Help is given to either active members, veterans, or any direct family member. If you become disabled while serving, the American Red Cross may help in customizing your home to meet your new needs. The Army's Wounded Warrior Project provides financial assistance for qualified soldiers, veterans, and their families for a variety of expenses. The goal with this program is to help any army member maintain their independence, through any means necessary, for in-home alteration and modification. These are just a few sources that can help. Before applying for any grant, check application deadlines, specific eligibility criteria, and other requirements.

Talk to your social worker and health-care team about obtaining information on these programs, public and private. The costs associated with making structural changes to your home could dramatically impact you and your family. Some programs are dedicated to providing financial assistance to amputees for assist devices and physical therapy treatments. Your social worker can help you gather information on local and national programs as part of your plan of going home. If things are tough financially, remember you have options. Look into reaching out to local charities and churches for possible assistance for financial help.

For most amputees taking the first steps in getting back into life can be daunting and even overwhelming. As a new amputee you will have to learn new methods for living and performing activities necessary in daily living. Basic activities of daily living involve everything from cooking, cleaning, getting dressed, bathing, paying bills, eating, and writing checks. These are things that most of us take for granted yet, now, as an upper or lower amputee, could prove to be a significant challenge. For example, if you have lost your writing hand or arm, writing checks, paying bills, and doing ordinary tasks around the house could prove challenging. Another example, if you're a lower amputee, getting in and out of the shower or maneuvering in the kitchen to prepare a meal could be problematic. Remember, be patient in these situations. Give yourself time to learn different ways to perform these kinds of daily tasks because it doesn't happen overnight. So start slow and build up by concentrating on every move you make. Living with limb loss, everything will now be a process of trial and error, and the challenge is figuring out ways to maneuver in ways that will work best for you. There is a learning curve, and you will need to train yourself in using new motor skills with the other healthy limb. Talk to your medical team for advice and work with your occupational therapist and prosthetist on solutions to help meet these daily challenges.

Whether you're an upper or lower limb amputee, getting dressed, buttoning shirts, putting on pants, and even tying shoelaces poses new and unforeseen difficulties. These simple acts require learning new skills, and over time you will figure it out. However, there are hundreds of videos on YouTube with helpful tips on how to maneuver many routine daily tasks. My good friend Julie J., a left-hand amputee, discovered many useful household items to help her with daily tasks. Here is what she suggests:

Dressing sticks: These devices are perfect for amputees with one hand or arm. They can be used to put on most anything, such as coats, shirts, vests, skirts, or pants. You can find them at most major medical supply retailers or on Amazon and other large online retailers.

Button aides: Buttoning shirts with two hands is simple. However, with one hand it's almost impossible. There is now new button-assistance technology such as different button aids and zipper-pull devices that are excellent. Having a device that incorporates both zipper and button help makes dressing easier and worry-free once again. Using these specifically designed products will help you button clothes, collars, and even cuff links. There are many new lines of "magnetically" designed shirts and pants that help you get dressed with ease.

Sock aids: These devices are designed to hold open a sock, making it easier to put on with one arm or hand. You can find them online or at any medical supplier.

Elastic shoelaces: There has been breakthrough technology in shoes for disabled people and amputees. Newly developed elastic shoelaces are now available, which are perfect for amputees missing an arm or hand. Elastic shoelaces allow an amputee to put on their shoes single-handedly without the need to tie the laces. Plus, they are great for lower limb amputees, removing the worry of untied shoelaces. These laces will enable the shoe to stretch open, making it effortless to place your foot inside, as well as a prosthetic, without the aid of a shoehorn.

One-handed belts: These newly designed belts are explicitly made to help anyone one-armed or -handed. They're designed to snap, slide, and secure, allowing you to put it on without hassle or stress.

One-handed nail clippers: Nail clippers were first invented in 1875. Over the centuries improvements to the original design have been made. Today, inventors have finally improved the design for a person missing an arm or hand. One-handed nail clippers are designed to sit on a flat surface while allowing you to cut your nails with one hand. It works by easily pressing down on the handle with either hand.

Hair dryer holder: Blow drying your hair is a normal, daily routine for most, but if you have one arm or one hand it can prove to be almost impossible. Today, there are specifically designed holders that keep hair dryers in place allowing for hands-free drying.

Experiment and embrace change by using your ingenuity to discover new ways to get yourself dressed. Human spirit is a powerful weapon. Most of us, when challenged or in danger, revert to primal instincts of survival, and taking care of yourself as an amputee isn't any different. You will soon learn new dressing skills. With the right tools and accessories, these daily activities do not have to be a dreaded event. The challenge is relearning everything you've learned in the past and approaching these tasks from a new perspective. Using technology to assist in daily living, along with your ingenuity and willpower, will give you newfound freedom as an amputee that will last your lifetime.

If you are a lower or upper limb amputee, bathing and using the bathroom may prove challenging. Everything from transferring up and off of the toilet with or without an assistive device to getting out of the shower are factors you must consider. Cleansing yourself properly as an upper or lower limb amputee could be troublesome. Relearning these skills is the only way to adapt and accomplish these tasks daily. Find safe ways to transfer in and out of the shower or bathtub by using specially designed transfer boards, and bathe safely with low-profile shower stools. Place shampoos and soap in easy to reach areas in your shower, and use back scrubbers and sponges to clean hard-to-reach areas of your body. Make things easier by keeping your towels and accessories in accessible places. Remember, as you start learning, if you have to ask for help, do not hesitate to seek it from a trusted family member. With practice, you will discover ways and adapt to doing it alone. It will take patience, but always trust your instinct. If you feel unsafe, then you probably are. So keep safety in the bathroom at the top of the list

EASY HOME MODIFICATIONS

One of the easiest things that will help the transition to home is making simple modifications to your house. If your loved one is a lower limb amputee, moving furniture out of the way, preparing the bathrooms for safe usage, and making utensils and food easier to access can help ease the transition from hospital to home. Remember, check for cables, cords, wires, or rugs, and remove clutter that could be troublesome to navigate around. You may find that your home isn't ready for you. If you are a lower limb amputee, you could have trouble reaching items on higher shelves, going up and down stairs, or maintaining balance in snow, grass, ice, sand, and even gravel. The family will need to make the necessary modifications as you transition from wheelchair to a new prosthesis. Check all entrances, doorways, exits, and floors for clearance and proper width. Consider changing existing doorknobs to levers and install indoor and outdoor motion-sensor lights. Examine the floors because if they are made of wood or vinyl, they may be slippery. Look at your kitchen as you may need to make some temporary changes and minor adjustments to cabinets and shelves. Install 180-degree hinges that allow cabinets to open easily and wide. Move everything needed to lower cabinets for easy access. This is helpful advice if your loved one is in a wheelchair.

For upper extremity amputees there are many modifications that can be helpful and necessary around the home. An easy one is to have straws for drinks, so you do not have to put down your eating utensil while dining. Install an automatic shampoo dispenser in the shower. For bathing, look for a long-handled body scrubber that will easily reach those hard-to-access parts of your body. Shower stools, flex shower heads and bathing accessories are always handy. When it comes to teeth brushing and toothpaste, purchase a specially designed dispenser that allows the sound hand to squeeze and dispense the toothpaste onto the toothbrush. Basic grooming for men and women, such as clipping nails, could be problematic when you only have one hand. There are specially designed one-handed suction nail clippers that help in getting the job done. Hair brushing can be done easily by installing a brush-holding and hair dryer stand that allows your loved one to brush with one hand and hold the blow dryer in the other.

GETTING AROUND INSIDE YOUR HOME

Depending on the architecture and design of your home, going home after limb loss could be frightening from a safety standpoint. Every home is different, and with every home, there are underlying aspects of your home that need to be addressed. Your living situation, overall, should be assessed for safety measures and plan for the best outcome. Talk with your hospital social worker or health-care patient services coordinator about what to expect when going home. Most of these professionals will provide helpful and insightful suggestions to help you prepare the home's interior and exterior for your return.

James D., an amputee friend who lost his right leg below the knee, told me that he and his wife wrote a direct homecoming plan before he was released to go home. "We knew it would be a few weeks before I returned home," James said, "so we took that time to figure it out." The plan allowed his wife to get things in order before James came home.

Modifications and adjustments will be necessary when you return home, and if you are a lower limb amputee, these are major decisions for you and your family. In the beginning, most alterations will be made to accommodate wheelchairs, walkers, or even knee scooters. If you are an upper limb amputee, modification to light fixtures, lamps, and electrical wall outlets may be necessary to help make your adjustment to home easier, daily tasks manageable, and your life easier.

Handrails and stair railings: Installing handrails or grab bars on any step inside and outside of your home may be necessary during the first weeks of recovery. This modification is not permanent yet can be helpful for both lower and upper limb amputees to make the adjustment to home life more manageable. Rails may be installed in bathrooms, around toilets, and in and around showers or bathtubs.

Outdoor lighting: Being able to see at night is an essential consideration for any amputee. Darkness affects balance and visibility, which could cause a hazard of falling and additional injury. If necessary, install outdoor lighting that can consist of solar-powered walkway lights, wheelchair ramp outdoor lights, and dusk-to-dawn lights. Set these motion-sensor lights around doors and garages for easy accessibility.

Bathroom accessories and accessibility: Bathroom accessories and accessibility need to be taken into serious consideration. Remember, your goal is to be as independent as soon as possible, and bathrooms must be addressed with safety in mind. Evaluate your bathrooms and make a list of any necessary adjustments to accommodate your specific amputation. Here are a few easy tips to help you in the bathroom:

- Liquid soap, with pump dispenser
- Nonslip mats for showers
- Sturdy shower stools
- Flexible hand-held shower head
- Lower shelves for towels and supplies
- Walk-in shower installed
- Grab bars next to the toilet and shower
- Simple night-light

Simple modifications such as these will provide a sense of security and peace of mind, along with keeping you safe. Feeling comfortable and secure at home is one of the first steps that will help in a quicker overall recovery.

Bedroom accessibility: If you are a lower limb amputee using a wheelchair or assistive device, depending on how your bedroom is designed, there are simple things you need to do to allow safe and easy access. Move any unnecessary furniture, loose rugs, clutter, wires, and electrical cords from your path for easy access in and out. Here are a few suggested items that could make your life easier in your bedroom during your recovery:

- Touch lamp
- Pull-string light fixtures
- Grab bars or poles
- More extended cell phone charging cables

- Transfer boards (wheelchairs and assistive devices)
- Extra accessories (plastic urinals, walking devices, flashlight, batteries, candles, lighter)
- Hang clothing lower for easy access

Kitchen accessibility: The kitchen is the most visited room in the house, and without planning, getting around that room for an upper or lower limb amputee can be a difficult challenge. Here are a few essentials to help you make your life easier in the kitchen throughout your recovery:

- Use the existing lower cabinets to store utensils and supplies.
- Store heavier foods such as jars and cans lower to alleviate heavy lifting if you are an upper amputee.
- Use your kitchen table for food prep instead of high countertops.
- Install grab bars to help you have the leverage to reach things and lift yourself to reach items from a seated wheelchair position.
- Place any essential and favorite foods on lower tiered shelves within your refrigerator.

Recognize the importance of preparing your home for a smooth transition from hospital to home. Remember, your family and friends are there to support you. Use their help to stay on track, and do not hesitate to ask for help if you need it. Please talk to your occupational therapist or local social worker about your home along with any specific and individual needs. Don't underestimate safety as a huge part of your recovery because preparing your home to make you safe as you adjust back into home life is crucial to your recovery. Recovery is virtually impossible if you feel unsafe within an unstable environment. These factors alone will cause undue stress, frustration, and, most of all, an unhappy new life. Strategic planning and assistance are critical factors for a safe and happy return home.

Managing Pain and Phantom Pain

> Without pain, there would be no suffering, without suffering we would never learn from our mistakes. To make it right, pain and suffering is the key to all windows, without it, there is no way of life.
>
> —Angelina Jolie

$\mathscr{I}$n the sixteenth century, French military surgeon Ambroise Paré was the first person to discover the phenomenon of phantom pain that followed amputation. In 1871, Paré, discovering that many amputee soldiers could still feel their missing limbs, coined the term "phantom limb." However, phantom pains differ from the actual physical pain you will experience after amputation. Understanding what you are experiencing is essential in your recovery. Pain profiles of amputees are complex and include nociceptive and neuropathic pain episodes. The medical description for nociceptive pain is the discomfort derived from any physical harm or damage to the body. The pain is acute, which means it resolves and feels better as the body heals. Nociceptive pain could be described as anything from arthritis to irritation from a sports injury or from a dental procedure. Neuropathic pain is different. It derives from damage to the nervous system and is the body's response to the ongoing damage through "misfirings" in the nervous system. Neuropathic pain happens even when the missing part of your body still receives existing nerve signals from the brain and they don't know where to go. When an amputate experiences these various neuropathic events, we commonly call them "phantom pains."

Differentiating between the two types of pain makes pain management challenging. We are human, and pain is one thing we all do our best to avoid. Still, limb loss brings varying degrees of pain that are virtually impossible to escape. Medications will help in being comfortable, yet, eventually, there is a time to endure and face what is hurting you. Pain is subjective, and you are the only one who knows the degree of pain you are feeling. Make sure to speak up and tell your doctor or others where the pain is and its degree of discomfort. Recognizing the level of pain is the only way to receive the right amount of treatment. After the amputation, your pain will intensify and eventually subside to manageable levels. Nevertheless, the pain could be so uncomfortable that it will be difficult to concentrate or relax. Sleep may become difficult from the pain, which can make it hard to function normally. Pain can affect your mood and even lead to bouts of depression, frustration, or make you feel overwhelmed and out of control.

Remember, don't be afraid to ask for pain medication to help you cope. Many amputees say the pains never subside and they need certain medications to help ease it. There are specific medications that can help treat phantom pains, including antidepressants, anticonvulsants (that treat epilepsy and neuropathy, for example), and other medicines like ketamine and beta blockers (that treat high cholesterol and the heart, for example). Antidepressants including Celexa, Lexapro, and Zoloft, for example, are used to treat phantom limb pain because they increase the level of serotonin in the brain, which when released attach (uptake) to other nerve receptors, stimulating other nerves causing less phantom pain. The only thing to be careful of when taking these drugs is to be fully aware of their side effects.

When you feel phantom pains, no matter the level, tell your doctor so treatment can begin early to prevent prolonged durations of them. Another amputee friend, Charles T., told me he had the hardest time coming forth to his doctor about phantom pain. He felt intimidated and shy about talking to his doctor or anyone else about what he was experiencing. However, once he did, Charles said it amazed him that his doctor knew exactly what he was talking about and describing. Your doctor is no stranger to the phantom pain situation either, so do not be afraid to speak up and let them know. Phantom pains are commonplace among the amputee community; even so, there isn't any shame in asking your doctor for necessary pain relief from them. Managing the pain during recovery is essential for emotional stability, and along with emotional support, pain medications help to promote fewer ongoing phantom pain symptoms. Yet with the pain you feel, be honest with yourself and your health-care team. If a medication isn't working or is causing severe side effects, let someone know. This way, they can change the drug to better suit your condition.

They can also treat pain management with the use of nonnarcotic pain medication. These types of medications are used as an effective method of treatment with fewer risks of adverse side effects. Nonnarcotic medications such as acetaminophen, ibuprofen, naproxen sodium, and others do not lead to addiction. When taking these drugs for pain, it is good advice to elevate your limb for effective blood flow and use isolated ice packs. Elevating the limb reduces any pressure points and slows blood flow, allowing you to rest and be more comfortable. If your pain only fades and does not entirely go away, these nonnarcotic medications should help to get over any pain hurdle.

Rating your pain may seem not important, but it is vital to your overall care and recovery. The nurses and staff should routinely evaluate your pain because your doctor uses that information to gauge if the prescribed pain treatment is working and in determining if you are receiving the correct dosage of medication. Varying pain scales are used in different hospitals around the country. One of the most common is the "FACES" pain management system. The level of pain, 0–10, is described by an illustrated facial expression, with 0 having no pain and 10 having the worst pain imaginable. Even though this system may not be 100 percent accurate, it is necessary to allow the proper pain treatment and course of action for your health-care team.

Narcotic pain medications treat varying levels of pain and, depending on your situation, they will be given either intravenously (IV) or orally. When administered through an IV, the patient can self-administer the medicine through a patient-controlled analgesia (PCA) pump. The medicine is administered when necessary by the patient. PCAs are closely monitored, yet convenient because when pain hits, all the patient has to do is push a button, allowing it to enter the bloodstream.

This brings up an important topic: safety and control of the medicines. High-dose drugs called opiates could cause significant damage to organs, form addiction, cause sickness, and even death. These drugs contain synthetic chemicals similar to those in opium. With prolonged use, the effects of opiates, including oxycodone or OxyContin, have been noted to result in adverse effects on the brain, which lead to irreparable damage. Therefore, opiates are administered in limited quantities and through strictly monitored dosages to avoid addiction and reliance. Codeine is labeled as a class of medication known as opiate analgesics, which can be administered in capsule, liquid, or tablet form. OxyContin and codeine are strictly regulated in the United States and are considered by law to be Schedule II narcotics. They are effective in treating pain by modifying how your nervous system reacts and responds to it. Receptors in the brain bond with the codeine and dull nerve endings. Although these drugs are effective in relieving pain, they do not help in speeding up the recovery period. Codeine, compared to other high-potency opioids like OxyContin and heroin, has a lower risk rating for dependency and addiction. Yet overall, it is still considered an addictive drug and should not be taken for long durations.

Most amputees experience acute pain (warning) and chronic pain (long-lasting) deriving from four different regions of the brain through our nervous system. To address this they have found that simple meditation can change these four areas of the brain to relieve both acute and chronic pain for amputees. All regions and areas of the brain are affected by meditation, and while proven effective, it doesn't entirely alleviate chronic pain. Meditation helps your brain reset, build stamina, and increase tolerance to the pain, allowing you to cope with it. Meditation is a way to control your mind and sensory receptors, including sound, sight, and pain, which is something we all experience.

There are many hospitals across the country that provide alternative therapies for pain management besides drugs and meditation. For amputees, there are various techniques, including acupuncture, aromatherapy, relaxation, massage, and music listening. These techniques have been useful in helping many amputees overcome their pain without medication or narcotic drugs. If this variety of techniques appeals to you and is something you would like to take part in, talk to your doctor or a health-care team professional about availability and how to get involved.

As mentioned previously, when a part of someone's body is lost, like an arm, hand, fingers, or leg, there is a high probability of experiencing pain in the missing limb. This pain is known as phantom limb syndrome (PLS). When experienced for the first time, phantom pains are unnerving. More than 80 percent of amputation patients report phantom pains either immediately after surgery or at later stages of their recovery. Phantom limb pain can show up when you least expect it. Changes in the patient's brain and damage to the nerves causes phantom limb pain. Neuroscientist V. S. Ramachandran researched phantom limb pain in the early 1990s and discovered and theorized that the pains were not from the nerves themselves but created directly within the brain. Ramachandran's theory concluded that after the limb is amputated, the portion of the brain assigned to that limb becomes frantic for sensations. In a frenzy and search for the nerve signals the brain generates the phantom pain signals causing phantom limb pain.

CAUSES OF PHANTOM PAINS

Phantom pains have been studied for centuries, and the direct causes remain inconclusive. Dr. Ramachandran touted the brain was the cause and not the stump or nerves. Although some medical professionals believe postamputation pains are a direct link to existing psychological problems, this doesn't seem to be the complete case. Medical experts have since discovered that phantom pain sensations originate through the connection of both the brain, nerves, and the spine.

When losing a limb through a traumatic event or accident, the limb is removed abruptly, and your brain doesn't have time to process the loss. The immediate loss makes your brain desperately search for connections that are now lost between the lost limb and your brain. The brain never stops signaling the nerves, hitting those that are no longer there, causing mild to severe phantom pains. This brain activity creates a roadblock of tangled nerves, causing the phantom pain that you are experiencing. Remember, as an amputee, you may continue to experience these phantom pains the rest of your life. They may fade and subside over time, yet be aware they could return now and again as your brain continues to map new nerve routes within your body. Phantom pains get better as your body continues to repair itself. The good news is that many amputees do not have to undergo any treatment for them.

PHANTOM PAIN SYMPTOMS

Although everyone experiences different physical pains, including headaches, earaches, toothaches, and stomach aches, phantom pains could arrive with varying intensity best described as throbbing, burning, aching, or cramping. Phantom pains have even been described by other amputees as:

- Jolts of electric shock
- Jabbing
- Sharp and stabbing
- Hot or burning pains
- Shooting pains
- Needles and pin pricks
- Crushing or squeezing pain
- Twisting and throbbing

Immediately after my surgery, my first phantom pains felt as if my toes were being crushed into my leg. After researching the topic, I discovered I was not alone. Phantom pains could feel like crushing and throbbing sensations, hot in temperature, tingly movement along with pressure, itchiness, and vibration. You may experience:

- Movement in the limb
- Telescoping (feelings of the limb getting longer or shorter)
- Temperature (hot or cold)
- Pressure or tugging
- Crushing
- Vibration
- Tingling and itching

Maybe you have experienced these types of phantom pains? If so, they are considered normal. Many amputees say they haven't experienced any phantom pains or have trouble distinguishing actual pain from phantom pains. I am on my fourth anniversary of being an amputee, and still every day, I experience a phantom sensation. I have come to terms with the phenomena and have now recognized how to differentiate physical stump pain from phantom limb pain. As you move through your recovery, you will be able to distinguish, understand, and cope with phantom pain and sensations. Be patient.

"Sometimes I have sudden pain like bolts of lightning, and it hurts," Timothy J., a new right-leg amputee, said while I visited him in the hospital. And like Timothy, I still experience these jolts of pain, yet over time, they have calmed down and are not fiery or sharp as they once were. Even today, some sensations lead me to believe my foot is still there. Often, I kind of welcome these feelings. Why? Because they remind me of younger days when my limbs were strong, intact, and healthy.

PHANTOM SENSATIONS

In 2019, a study was published on phantom pains. A team of researchers from New York University, Bielefeld, Germany, and the University of Hamburg published their findings of what defines, differentiates, and characterizes phantom sensations. Lead researcher, Professor Tobias Heed, wrote, "The limitations of the previous explanations for how and where our brain processes touch become apparent when it comes to individuals who have had parts of their bodies amputated or suffer from neurological diseases."[1] He continued, "To this day, scientists know surprisingly little about how the human brain processes the sensation of touch." In the article Professor Heed wrote, "People who have had a hand, or a leg amputated often report phantom sensations in these limbs." He also observed and noted, "But where exactly does this false perception come from?"[2]

Researchers have discovered how the brain processes the sense of touch by forming a road map within the brain to where the nerve signals are coming and going. The parts of our body, like the feet, legs, arms, and hands, are specific destinations on the configured road map. This makes us all the same when it comes to our brains and phantom sensations being a standard occurrence. Even though the explanation of phantom pains is still a mystery among the scientific community, the consensus is that phantom sensations are the brain continuing the process of signaling the limb or limbs that are no longer there. Because of the abruptness of amputations, the mind needs time to accept the trauma. During this time the rerouting of nerve signals simulates the strange sensations and tricks the brain to thinking that the missing body part is still there.

Unlike phantom pains, phantom sensations are, in most instances, not painful. Still, they can make you feel sad or depressed because they resemble sensations of actually moving your missing limb, stirring up memories that cause an unexpected outburst of emotions.

I believe that amputation qualifies as a stressful period of your life. Even emotional stress can cause the onset of phantom sensations. Phantom sensations could evoke confusing and even painful emotions when the sensations remind you of when the limb was still there. These emotions could make you feel sadness, grief stricken, depressed, or even angry. Remember, it is normal to feel these kinds of emotions, and there isn't anything wrong with you. Although these sensations fade over time, even so if the phantom sensations persist, seek help. Talk to your doctor or professional therapist for guidance.

KINETIC SENSATIONS

"I woke up and felt as if my missing limb was twisted and it hurt bad!" Tina H. said during a peer visit. Phantom sensations could cause mild to severe pain because it may feel as if the missing limb is in an awkward position. These are called kinetic sensations and are often referred by other amputees as "spasms." Tammy, a left-leg below-the-knee amputee, once told me, "I felt as if my left leg was twisted, and it felt as I had sprained my ankle." Other amputees I have spoken with reported experiencing feelings of their missing arms and legs as tingly, as if the limb had "fallen asleep." These kinetic sensations can be freaky and painful, and if you experience them, just relax and simply move your limb in your mind. Think of a specific movement to free your missing limb through imaginary motion. In most instances, the simple imaginary movement will make the phantom sensations go away.

Emotional stress can also trigger kinetic sensations along with physical pressure on the remaining limb. Stress can prompt stronger kinetic sensations, and they could feel itchy, tingly, needlelike, and/or feel like dull or intense pressure. These sensations could even feel as if someone is touching you or as something lying on your missing limb. Usually, kinetic sensations don't hurt but are mostly irritating, distracting, and even borderline annoying. Be patient, as you will adapt and build tolerance to these sensations. There are specific methods you can practice that will reduce kinetic sensations through desensitizing your residual limb. If you need help in this area, please speak to your doctor.

With phantom pains the problem is the barrier between physical and phantom feelings because, initially, it is challenging to distinct which is which. This makes it challenging and even harder to relieve with proper medication. The good news is that often these sensations will subside over time without using pain medications.

MIRROR THERAPY

Neuroscientist Vilayanur S. Ramachandran was the first to discover the use of a mirror box to treat phantom limb pain. Mirror therapy, successful with a multitude of amputees, led Dr. Ramachandran to continue the use and further study correlating brain function and phantom pains along with expanding his work of mirror neurons. Mirror therapy uses visualization through reflection of your healthy limb. The reflection sends images of the healthy limb, "tricking the brain" into believing the missing limb is still there. The technique satisfies the brain's continuous search for the missing limb, reverting the nerve signals, thus relieving symptoms of phantom pains. Results published in *The New England Journal of Medicine* in 2007, show that mirror therapy was effective for reducing phantom pain after four weeks of regular practice.

HOW TO PERFORM MIRROR THERAPY

- Use a standard mirror, preferably a longer one for leg amputation or a shorter one for arm and hand amputations.
- If you have an arm or hand limb loss, you can position the mirror on a table, and for a leg amputation, the use of the floor, sofa, or bed is ideal.
- Position the mirror with either the missing arm or leg hidden behind the mirror.
- Therapy begins when the mirror reflects the healthy arm or leg. By visualizing the healthy limb where the missing limb is, the

brain starts the process of programming that an amputation hasn't happened.
- Always make sure the mirror is stable so your mind can fully concentrate on the reflective image during the treatment.
- While viewing the reflection, make small incremental movements so the brain registers the movements supporting the therapy.

For the best results perform this mirror therapy for twenty to thirty minutes per day.

COGNITIVE BEHAVIORAL THERAPY

Many amputees across the United State have reported success from cognitive behavioral therapy and relief from phantom pains. This method of treatment is implemented to change the thought process of how an amputee thinks about the pain—and themselves. More than 30 percent of amputees are affected by bouts of depression caused by low self-esteem and negative perceptions of their body. Therefore, many amputees remained in self-isolation because losing a limb is difficult to come to terms with mentally, and many amputees find it challenging to adjust to the loss. This is normal not only because of an obvious loss of a limb but also the harshness of the reality of loss of motor function, self-image, career, and even relationships. Cognitive-behavioral therapy has been used effectively to combat these negative feelings. It can also help with the symptoms of post-traumatic stress disorder experienced by many amputees. How we perceive ourselves is significant, and many amputees encounter negative body image shock leading to high anxiety and even sexual dysfunction in men and women. Cognitive-behavioral therapy can help address these mental and emotional challenges and hopefully ease or avoid bouts of depression. Still, it will require working closely with your doctor and behavioral specialists to achieve the desired results. If you want to learn more about cognitive-behavioral therapy, talk to your doctor.

WARM TOWEL THERAPY

Often you can get relief from phantom pains or sensations by wrapping the area with a warm towel. The warmth of the towel is not only beneficial to circulation but it gently massages the pain area, stimulating the brain and nerves to cease sending pain signals. Warm towels can also help improve circulation leading to less pain and fewer occurrences of phantom pains.

MENTAL EXERCISE

Mental imaginary movement of your lost limb can help alleviate phantom pains or kinetic sensations. Simple exercises in your mind can bring excellent results. These imaginary movements of the missing limb start a positive mental change within your brain. By doing this regularly, your brain records the movement and stores them away to help reduce any pain. This exercise can help when you experience kinetic movements and pains where the missing limb feels as if it is a painful position. By imagining your missing limb moving in different motions, the pains should subside quickly.

SIMPLE TAPS

When you feel phantom pains, simply tap on the area to alleviate or reduce the sensations. The tapping sends reverse signals back to the brain, alerting it of the physical touch. Next, the brain receives the message, and the pain subsides and hopefully disappears.

SURVIVING AMPUTEE PAIN

I want to say that being an amputee has its great rewards, but it is difficult on many levels. Your recovery will be one of endurance, tolerance, and a show of heart to get your life back to normal. Pain will be intense, yet each day you will get stronger and more tolerant as your body heals, gradually making the pain subside. Once your pain is manageable, you will become comfortable, thus helping you overall to recuperate.

Living as an amputee has a definite learning curve. Everything from walking, standing, and even eating can be a major challenge. Coping with what is in front of you will be difficult and one of the hardest things you will ever endure. However, the good news is that you will adapt and your life will vastly improve. The key is to remain strong, steadfast, and most of all—never, ever quit. Keep pushing yourself.

Remember, while in recovery your only mission is to do everything within your power to cope, manage, accept, and handle the pain. It's okay if you need to work through the pain with the help of medications or other alternative methods for a little while. Keep in mind that pain is not always physical because it can appear as hurtful, deep-seated emotions. As a new amputee, you will encounter both physical pain and/or emotional pain. They are part of the challenges you must overcome in getting yourself back to living a healthy life. Believe in yourself, pick yourself up, seek help if needed. Your goal is to return to the life that you love—and want to live.

• 8 •

Your Physical Recovery

Courage is being scared as hell but saddling up anyway.

—John Wayne

RECOVERY: DURATION AND EXPECTATIONS

$\mathcal{A}$s of this writing it has been four years since I lost my left leg below the knee. As I look back on my limb loss journey, it has been a strange and wondrous ride, slow and lasting, yet seemingly quick and eye-opening. When I started my recovery, one of the fundamental questions I had was how long it would be before I could walk again. "It could be up to a year before you're back up on your feet," my doctor said. I'll never forget that day because after I heard those words, I felt lost and deflated, and his words took the wind out of my sails. Still other doctor friends told me it would be a year, or even two, in physical therapy and psychological healing. I admit those words stung, but I'm stubborn and decided that I would not listen to all the naysayers. I had the desire, the will, the drive, and the heart to get myself back up, and I knew I was going to fight, work hard, and walk again. You can, too.

Still, I stuggled with coming to terms with the fact that my life was changed forever. It was hard to accept, but I still had a life to live. Being stuck in a wheelchair or holed up in a corner for the world to forget was something I just could not do. Everyone that knows me understands one critical variable: I am a fighter, and I never give up. There wasn't any way I was going to let a missing leg stop me. Don't misunderstand: I was afraid of the unknown. I was scared as hell of what I was facing;

the uncertainty and the challenges were all a massive mystery to me. I was headed into this blind, not knowing what my recovery journey looked like or what to expect. The only thing I knew was that I wasn't going to quit. This personal oath and faith in myself were the driving forces I held onto to get me through. I attacked the situation with all my strength and used the burning desire to get back up, to stand, to walk again. Walking upright was at the frontline of the fight of my life. My happiness, joy, and feeling whole again depended upon me accomplishing this goal. It was there, in front of me, ripe for the taking. Holding onto my determination, I believe my recovery efforts could be considered living proof of the true human spirit.

However, as you can see, your attitude and mindset play a critical part in how well and how fast you recover. Depending on your health condition, your recovery time and duration will vary. A positive mindset is crucial to getting started on the right path. Having the wrong attitude will slow your progress and be a major detriment to your overall recovery. Losing a limb is hard enough, and your approach mentally will make the complete night-and-day difference. I have met amputees with low self-esteem, who, in their own way, were holding themselves back from moving forward. I think it is incredibly sad when an amputee cannot see the light of their lives, and instead of hope they see bleakness and despair, which slows their recovery to a sluggish crawl. No doubt these are hard things to face. We are all human, but negative thinking and the physical challenges hang on hard and become difficult to shake. They will affect your physical healing, slow you down mentally, hinder mobility, and even attack your emotional recovery. President Theodore Roosevelt wrote, "Believe you can and you're halfway there." He was right. It takes belief in yourself and a strong, positive mindset. A poor attitude could make your recovery even more grueling than it needs to be.

Every one of us is guilty, when we experience negative things, to instinctively want to run away. Limb loss isn't any different. When you experience pain, human nature makes us want to get away, remove ourselves from what hurts or puts us in harm's way. This is science at its best and our human brain, doing what it does best by seeking ways to not work so hard and take the easy way out. Our human response to anything contrary is fight-or-flight; in adverse situations our brain naturally sends cortisol to the muscles of our body, inflicting the flight reaction from anything hurtful, painful, or seemingly harmful. Once you overcome this flight response and push your mind and body to forge through what hurts, things will drastically change. It is simply mind over matter that will make it happen. As you work through your recovery, push yourself with all that you have, be strong in mind and spirit, and don't go backward. Keep moving forward or you may face a dismal recovery defeat. Remember, a thriving and successful recovery is within your reach—the choice is entirely up to you.

Medically and physically, on average, depending whether your amputation is lower extremity or upper extremity, your recovery could be approximately two to three months. Upper limb amputees will have shorter hospital stays and recovery times. Once again, how quickly you recover depends on your attitude, which will have a direct influence on how long you're in the hospital. Regrettably, I have witnessed amputees remaining in the hospital for more than a year or more, all because of their negative mindset and attitude. Your recovery time depends upon listening to your doctors and taking care of yourself. Everything is based on how seriously you want to get your life back and what you want to do. No matter your situation, seize the moment, work hard, believe in yourself, and do everything within your power to get your life back. However, if you are a lower extremity amputee, prepare yourself for an extreme amount of hard, physical work in learning to walk again and being mobile. Your trained therapist should introduce new recovery exercises to keep you on track with goals to be met. During recovery training you will be challenged, and it will be scary as the initial recovery sessions will comprise daily physical therapy with different training devices to regain your mobility. This is where the tough get going. Be prepared as the training could be grueling and challenging, with possible intense pain. Don't let it get to you because this is where a strong mindset comes into play. Be a warrior and fight. You must be strong inside and out, and push yourself beyond the limit while fighting through the pain. Keep telling yourself, "You can do it."

Limb loss is not only extremely hard on us physically but is more so emotionally. The emotional impact of limb loss, at first, cannot be measured as amputation is forever life changing. There isn't a way of getting around it because every amputee, young or old, deals with the deep-rooted physical and emotional aspects of limb loss. The only varying degree is emotional pain can happen at different times throughout your limb loss life. As you know, physical pain hits almost immediately, all on varying levels, but emotions may come into play initially or later on. Emotions are tricky as they can appear unexpectedly weeks, months, or even years later. Emotions are subtle, but some amputees experience physical pain and emotional trauma simultaneously. This is what I experienced. When this happens it makes for a tough as hell situation. Understand that your amputation will be a daily reminder that something isn't the same and at first could spark an onslaught of confusing emotions. These are all factors every amputee faces and one of the primary reasons it takes strength and willpower to overcome the emotional and physical pain. Remember, the battle you're fighting is not all yours as others have met the challenge, and you will, too. You are not alone.

Since we're talking about the two significant aspects of limb loss, the physical and emotional side, one crucial factor to recognize is that you are the only person who knows sole limitations. How much time you need to recover isn't on a time clock. Push yourself, work hard, and seek help, but do it at the pace that is comfortable for you. It is not a race. This is your time, and no matter what everyone says, take the necessary time you need to fully recover. Now, I am not saying to take forever or quit on yourself. You know your body and your limitations so be kind to yourself. Don't compare yourself to others. Allow yourself to heal. Be mindful of your physical and emotional healing because powerful emotions can add undue anxiety and stress, keeping you from a full recovery.

One critical aspect to consider during this time is your family and loved ones. They are going through this alongside you, and everything about your recovery affects your family, whether or not you see it. They are experiencing and seeing the consequences of your limb loss firsthand in their lives. Recovery, overall, includes healing for not only you but your family as well. Take the time to grieve along with your family, and don't be afraid to talk with them about how you feel. During this time, a caring friend, a trusted loved one, or mental health professional could make the difference. There isn't anything wrong with talking openly about your feelings and what you're going through. Being open about your experiences, feelings, and emotions can help you and your family lead a happier and prosperous new life.

PHYSICAL THERAPY OVERVIEW

A few days after my surgery, my back became sore from lying down, so I moved around to sit on the side of the bed. As I swung my right leg around, the momentum pulled me forward and pulled me off the bed, straight down onto the floor. The fall jarred me, and I thought I had damaged myself. Nurses ran into the room, and a male nurse ran over to me.

"Lift yourself," he said, holding out his arm.

"I can't!" I grimaced, looking up from the floor. "My right leg is too weak. I'm not ready to lift my body."

"Sure you can," he said. He placed his foot sideways and planted it firmly. "Now, push yourself up," he said. I put my right foot up against his and pushed. I used every ounce of my arm strength along with what little strength in my right leg to get myself back into the bed. At first I was angry and couldn't believe what he had done to me. But as I sat there, safely back in the bed, I realized he had just given me my first lesson of the hard work required to get myself back up on my feet. It would not be easy, but with tough love, he showed me I could do it.

Physical therapy is an essential part of your recovery. If you are an upper extremity amputee, you will, in most cases, work with physical and occupational therapists to help you adapt to your new prosthetic or learn to not use one. Losing a limb involves a massive adjustment to the immediate changes happening to your body, and these changes can be painful and often demanding to cope with. A physical therapist, skilled in working one-on-one with amputees, can help you overcome these immediate challenges. They can help you adjust by developing specific strategies, along with unique exercises, to bolster your body as you go through your journey to recovery.

With lower limb amputees, physical therapy, along with getting mobile, is vital to maintaining strength and good optimal health after limb loss. As a lower extremity amputee, you will be introduced to various devices that will assist you in getting active. Once acclimated, the key is to push and fight through the pain by getting up and using the device as soon as you can. Being active and exercising through your recovery will boost morale and encourage optimal health, spirit, and mind. Newfound mobility is empowering and uplifting as your body adjusts to the loss. This extra attention to yourself, spirit and mind, will help you recover as soon as possible because physical activity provides significant benefits and offers substantial advantages in strengthening and supporting your psychological condition. Some immediate and long-term benefits you will experience by staying active after surgery include:

- Improved cardiovascular health (lung, heart, and respiratory system health)
- Psychological improvements and benefits
- Increased core strength
- Strengthened balance
- Gained muscle strength and stamina

Remember, never attempt activity without help until you are confident and ready. Consult your doctor and physical therapist about your specific situation to determine if you are healthy and ready to get moving. Before getting started, discuss a plan of activity with your healthcare team. Physical activity could help reduce your risk for heart attacks, strokes, or any other type of cardiovascular disease along with diabetes. Initially, as a lower limb amputee, being confined to a wheelchair or bed causes major inactivity and possible weight problems. Getting active will strengthen your endurance and help in losing weight, which is critical in aiding you with balance and other prominent issues. Moving and being active creates a leaner body mass that will help in every area of your life, especially with diabetes and cardiovascular diseases. Being up and mobile early on will also improve psychological aspects that may be occurring. Feeling better improves your self-esteem, outlook on your body image, and acceptance of your amputation, thus improving your quality of life.

Overall, activity and exercise can provide much-needed core strength and flexibility, making it easier to prepare for your prosthetic. Once you receive your prosthetic, you should undergo gait training. Core strength and balance are vital in gait training; as a lower limb amputee, it is essential to learn to walk with your prosthetic device. All the exercise and activity improve your stamina and memory muscle strength. As your muscle strength increases, the risk of falls and injuries reduces. As you work and get stronger, your recovery and daily activities become manageable with less fatigue and other difficulties.

GAIT TRAINING:
THE IMPORTANCE TO AN AMPUTEE (LOWER LIMB)

All lower limb amputees strive to get back up and walk again, and the primary goal is to walk upright and naturally and avoid walking off balance or with a "hitch." Gait training is essential in avoiding walking abnormally with a hitch. This intense yet therapeutic training is where you learn to stand and walk again by using bars and apparatuses designed to help you maneuver and practice with your prosthetic. They also design these training sessions to instill confidence, address fitting problems, and any balance issues when walking. Gait training also allows your health-care team to examine your step length, rate of speed, ease of motion, posture, and specific positioning of your limb/s as you step. Learning to stand and walk again will not be easy. I wish I could say otherwise. Getting back up and walking will be fraught with new challenges, yet the goal is to improve coordination and mobility while not depleting your entire energy reserves or over exerting yourself.

I cannot overemphasize essential gait training and the importance of the process. There will be intensive work ahead and you must be strong and ready to endure. Many new lower limb amputees do not know what to expect and believe walking again will be a breeze. Do not allow yourself to think physical therapy or training is unnecessary. As you recover and begin with your prosthesis, gait training, strength training, and physical therapy are critical elements for your life.

Depending on your specific health condition, rehabilitation and gait-training practice could endure for a few months. Routine gait training is necessary to allow for precise modifications so your gait will be stable, balanced, smooth, and safe. Remember, everyone is different, and how long it takes to train and relearn walking, building strength, and improving flexibility is up to you. Work with your health-care team and therapist, along with your prosthetist, to ensure you get the quality training for a successful recovery.

Daniel H. Wilson, robotic engineer and *New York Times* best-selling author of *Robopocalypse* (2011), said, "The goal for many amputees is no longer to reach a 'natural' level of ability but to exceed it, using whatever cutting-edge technology is available. As this new generation sees it, our tools are evolving faster than the human body, so why obey the limits of mere nature?"[1]

If you are an above-the-knee amputee, the challenge to walk again is even more intense. Learning the fundamentals of walking with an above-the-knee prosthesis will be a group undertaking and effort with your caregivers. Training will be intense as you learn to use adaptive prosthetic technology with your therapist and prosthetist. Above-the-knee prosthetics require walking and standing with two different joints: the knee and ankle. Along with this training you will learn balance and ambulation. This will be hard work and require you to remain steadfast, driven, and motivated to endure the stringent rehab process. Trust in yourself and your team to push you and know that your hard work will pay off. The specific training will help you walk again and move on with your life, enjoy your days, and get back to pursuing everything you want and dream to do. Work with your physical therapist on the specific activity plan of functional strength exercises to build movement along with obtaining stable balance. These practical exercises are designed to emulate your everyday movements to retrain your body and mind to move normally and rebuild coordination in specific muscles. A good physical therapist or certified personal trainer should understand the concepts of adaptive or inclusive fitness and create a plan of exercise specific for your needs.

INNER WORKINGS OF PHYSICAL THERAPY

Strength Training

Strength training will play an essential part in your recovery and could begin right after surgery and continue over weeks and months. Once your limb area is stable and healed, you can begin strengthening exercises, starting with floor exercises. They design these types of floor exercises to strengthen muscles in your remaining healthy limb to prepare for the bulk lifting and weight bearing in being mobile. A physical therapist should design a floor exercise regime specific for your health situation. The different activities will help develop strength in core areas to prepare for prosthesis training. Core training is essential in maintaining mobility of joints and building muscle mass and power in the weight-bearing remaining limb. Your healthy limb is now the main wheel on your mobility vehicle (body) and is the primary means to get you where you want to go.

Graded Motor Injury Therapy

I discovered graded motor injury therapy by accident. After my surgery, as I was coming out of anesthesia, my left leg was on fire with pain, and it felt as though my left toes had been "crushed" into my leg. I could feel my missing toes moving and wriggling, and I found the sensation startling but oddly empowering. It amazed me that my brain had the power to visualize my toes that weren't there any longer. I kept up the practice, and to this day I use the visualization method if I feel phantom pains to help my body and brain adjust to make myself more comfortable. Graded motor injury therapy is an effective treatment to help alleviate phantom pains by visualizing the movement of the missing limb. This type of therapy involves deep science of motor neurons and mirror neurons in your brain. The mirror neurons fire as you imagine the movement in your limb or when you watch another person move.

Through your recovery you will increase your mobility day by day. Yet remember, it is not a race. Embrace this time to do everything you can do and push yourself—but understand your limits. Work hard and over time your stamina will increase and improve. Don't hesitate to use every means necessary, such as crutches, walkers, or wheelchairs, to get mobile. Through it all, your full recovery entirely depends on you, your tenacity, and willpower to be active, mobile, and moving as soon as you can.

IV

THE EMOTIONAL RECOVERY

· 9 ·

Dealing with Grief and Depression

Character cannot be developed in ease and quiet. Only
through experience of trial and suffering can the soul be
strengthened, ambition inspired, and success achieved.[1]

—Helen Keller

$\mathcal{L}$imb loss is traumatic, and we can compare the grief it brings to
the same intense grief experienced when a family member dies. With
traumatic events, such as death or amputation, human nature makes us
extremely emotional. As you begin the journey of living with limb loss,
grief and depression can set in intensely within your life. C. S. Lewis, in
his book *A Grief Observed*, wrote, "The death of a beloved is an amputation" (2009). Limb loss can be more psychologically devastating than
death. Going through the emotional storm is challenging to describe
because the reality of the loss is intensified, even magnified, because
you are trying to make sense in your mind of the reality that you've lost
a physical part of you—and it is gone forever. This harsh awareness is
difficult to face because your life has now drastically changed forever,
with a newfound trajectory, met with firsthand challenges, with no way
to return to the way it was. Emotionally, all these factors can take their
toll and deeply affect your very being, especially in the beginning.

Grief and limb loss seem to be intertwined, having dramatic effects
on your life. Remember, no one experiences the same levels of grief or
feels the same emotions, so the grieving time is a personal experience
that only you alone can endure. Grief comes in stages with bouts of
feeling out of control, helpless, and even feeling worthless. There may
be times when you feel angry, hopeless, frustrated, confused, guilty, sad,

and even remorseful. All of these emotions can hit you one by one or at the same time, in one massive, hard, emotional punch. As part of your recovery, grieving begins with recognizing the emotions as they surface and accepting the situation. The emotional pain could leave you feeling damaged inside to the point you cannot do the things you enjoy. It can affect everything in your life such as hobbies, activities, relationships, work, taking part in sports, or even playing with your children. I visited my good friend Gary W., a right-leg below-the-knee amputee, a month after he lost his right leg from a bad work-related injury. Gary told me he felt he had missed not being able to see his kid play in his first Little League game. His amputation happened right before the season opener, and he was in the hospital and couldn't be there in person. "It was his first Little League game, and I hated missing it," he said. The good news was that his family used FaceTime so Gary could see his son play in real time. So there was hope, but the feelings of missing out and sorrow were strong for Gary. The problem is emotions happen and affect each of us to varying degrees, at unexpected times, and at different stages. Learning to manage this outpouring of emotions is critical, as is adapting to the changes affecting everything in your life. Every portion of your life will be affected, and what makes it so hard to handle is that most of the time, the changes are abrupt. There isn't a learning period or learning curve with grief. It's a do-or-die situation because the pain inside, mixed with the physical pain, can take its toll and hinder your overall recovery. Give yourself permission to grieve, let it go, let your heart and spirit heal, and allow yourself time to restore emotionally.

Elizabeth Kubler-Ross (2014), author of *On Death and Dying*, wrote, "The reality is that you will grieve forever. You will not 'get over' the loss of a loved one; you will learn to live with it. You will heal and you will rebuild yourself around the loss you have suffered. You will be whole again, but you will never be the same. Nor should you be the same, nor would you want to."

Limb loss is the same. I believe you never truly get over losing a limb; it merely becomes a part of your life. Emotional healing takes time and self-awareness as you learn to live with your amputation. Recovery truly arrives by teaching our minds and body to accept the change as the new normal. Thinking of your limb loss as an entirely "new you" is the best place to begin. Yet the challenge is getting to that acceptance place in your mind and spirit. I know how hard this battle is and still I know it can be won. The way to overcome is to take it one step at time and conquer it by recognizing the stages. Kubler-Ross (2014) identifies grief occurring in five specific stages:

1. Shock
2. Denial
3. Anger
4. Bargaining
5. Depression

Along with these five, researchers have uncovered two additional stages of grief: testing and acceptance.

Every one of us will experience the different stages of grief. They are felt universally, in all walks of life, yet strike at different times and in various ways. Still, only in recent years has the medical community recognized grieving as a serious factor of limb loss recovery. Grieving stages among amputees are now being studied because of the psychological and physical implications on overall recovery and quality of life. A healthy emotional recovery starts by educating yourself about the emotional stages and how each can affect your life. Being able to recognize the stages of grief will first help in understanding what to expect after your limb loss.

SHOCK

One of the initial stages of grief is shock. Experiencing shock is normal and an immediate coping mechanism after your limb loss. It's a way for you to comprehend the grief and disbelief of it. Losing a part of your body is traumatic, and shock can be extremely hard as your mind tries to cope with what has happened to your body. This reaction, shock, involves disbelief, making it impossible to comprehend the reality of your missing limb. During this stage the loss may appear devastating, even surreal, as if you are living in a bad dream—one you'll never wake up from. Most new amputees I speak to, when asked, say they feel lost and cannot concentrate on anything around them during this phase. Shock and feeling as if you are immersed in a bad dream, or nothing seems real, is a normal emotional process in response to shock and limb loss.

DENIAL

Susan Forward, author of *Toxic Parents; Overcoming Their Hurtful Legacy and Reclaiming Your Life* (2009), wrote that "Denial is the lid on our emotional pressure cooker: the longer we leave it on, the more pressure we build up. Eventually, that pressure is bound to pop the lid, and we have an emotional crisis."[2] The term "emotional crisis" is impactful, but viable, in your situation because shock and denial are both emotional locomotives burning out of control. Even though denial can be dangerous ground, experiencing it is commonplace because our minds are trying to absorb the situation and protect us from the immense pain. We can describe denial as part of the fight-or-flight protection mechanism of our inner selves. Our brains operate like a swinging pendulum and are constantly monitoring visual stimuli, either positive or negative. So with denial, your brain is on red alert by immediately opening and closing the gate, depending on how much emotional pain you are feeling. Emotional pain could skyrocket after limb loss, perhaps even more than you can handle, causing shutdown and complete denial.

Denial can be a long phase that leads to bouts of acute anxiety and stress. Anxiety is a complicated and painful emotion that causes feelings of fear of the unknown. Losing a part of your body could trigger this deep-rooted anxiety, unleashing obscure thoughts such as fear of loss of mobility, independence, love, finances, and even your life. Anxiety could also emerge as intense fear of never being able to physically function normally. Having anxiety could involve deeper fears such as death, chronic illness, severe disability, and losing everything in your life. Most anxiety episodes bring feelings of panic and dread, which could be emotionally debilitating. Mark Twain wrote, "Braveness is resistance to concern, mastery of panic—not absence of anxiety."[3] Anxiety is real and a roller-coaster of emotions causing even worse thoughts and feelings that can be scattered, disoriented, and disorganized. If you experience being tense, not being able to perform daily functions or taking care of your basic needs, such as eating, drinking, or even sleeping, please seek help from a medical professional.

Denial can trigger catastrophic thinking, which causes you to envision the worst outcome in everything in your life. Things can become extremely difficult if you start to believe there isn't any hope or things just don't matter any longer. After she lost both her legs in a tragic car accident, my amputee friend Marie W. told me she would lie awake at night and think of the most horrible things. One night she said she even planned her own funeral because she felt death was the only thing left and that her life was over. I know how Marie felt because after my limb loss I worried about my family, kids, career, and how I could support my family. Everything seemed hopeless, and worse—I felt worthless. If you're not careful, catastrophic thinking can consume and eat you away emotionally, leaving you drained and physically spent.

If you ever have these catastrophic thinking events, leaving you completely exasperated, don't hesitate and seek immediate help from someone. They could leave you not understanding everything that you're feeling and cause even more stress to your mind and body. The first step in these scenarios is acknowledging you need help, so seek professional guidance in dealing with these levels of emotional pain. The powerful, emotional battles are a real factor as you move through the various stages of grief. Yet handling these catastrophic thoughts is a significant progression in your recovery.

ANGER

Anger is one of the most prominent and challenging stages of grief. It is considered a primal emotion, yet society views it as a taboo because most of us are taught to suppress feelings of hostility, anger, or rage toward others. As a Certified Peer Visitor through the Amputee Coalition, I talk to many amputees going through the early stages of grief and often ask them if they ever feel angry. This seems to be a hard question for many to answer. Why? Because many amputees are angry yet afraid to let out what society says should be suppressed. Many amputees feel that displaying their anger shows weakness or gives the impression they want to hurt someone or themselves. Through my peer visits and my experience, I've seen that expressing anger is a necessary step in the process. Even though it may appear negative, openly conveying anger is a positive step in your overall recovery.

Allowing yourself to be angry is a critical step in the stages of grief. The reality is you have just lost a limb and have an exponential right to be angry. Anger arises because you will have questions without answers. And anger can escalate because losing a limb is confusing and hard to accept in the beginning. The key is to not let anger reach an out-of-control level. If you feel angry, find a place of solitude, be alone for a while, and let it out. Scream into a pillow, cry, squeeze something hard, but never attack someone out of anger because lashing out in fits of rage can irreparably damage relationships. Keep anger in control. In hindsight, you will realize that anger allowed you to move forward in your recovery.

I spoke to a new amputee James V., and after a friendly conversation he suddenly became silent. I asked him what was wrong. He told me he was embarrassed and felt as if something was wrong with him. "Other amputees around me seem angry" James said, "but, honestly, I am not. I just don't feel angry about it all, and I am doing my best to accept it and move on." These were simple yet profound words that spoke volumes to me. I knew then that James was probably experiencing other stages of grief and simply hadn't yet reached the anger stage. This is common. You may experience varies stages of grief other than anger. Still, not being angry isn't unusual or abnormal, but not expressing anger because of what others may think could present additional problems down the road. Be aware that suppressed anger can cause increased stress that could lead to heart issues, headaches, ulcers, and even drug or alcohol dependency. Remember, being angry about limb loss is valid and real. Releasing these feelings can provide a deep sense of relief and other healing properties. Getting through the anger phase is essential because no one wants to truly live angry for the rest of their lives and neither do you. Being angry makes your life and everyone around you miserable. If you discover your anger reaching out-of-control levels, seek help if needed, but let it out, free yourself, and open up to a whole new life ahead.

DEPRESSION

Depression during the grieving stage is one of the most common, yet one of the most critical, challenging, and painful stages of your recovery. Depression is where the tough gets tougher and, in most instances, hits most amputees with a vengeance. Depression is real, universal, widely experienced, and commonly appears once the reality of your limb loss takes hold of your life. Depression can show itself in many ways, for example, feeling hopeless, helpless, devastated, and even agony. However, depression is a sneaky emotion. It may emerge slowly, showing up as a lack of motivation, overeating, loss of appetite, solitude, drug use, or even insomnia. Depression may leave you feeling closed off or as if an invisible wall is in front of you that you are completely unable to climb or get over. If you are experiencing chronic depression or escalating emotional problems, seek professional help immediately. Depression, if left untreated, could lead to thoughts of suicide. Remember, there is help available. Volunteers at the National Suicide Prevention Hotline (1-800-273-8255) or online at www.suicidepreventionlifeline.org, are available and ready to help you through this traumatic time.

Depression has two distinct phases: worry and isolation. Have you ever found yourself worrying about family, friends, your career, or possibly money? Have you made the mistake of seeing no value in yourself? Do you take care of everyone around you except yourself, placing yourself dead last? If you answered yes, this could be considered clinical depression. The second phase of depression is feeling isolated and closed off. Have you ever felt like you want to be alone all the time? Do you feel better away from people and society? Maybe you feel as if you don't want to talk to anyone around you? We also identify these feelings as having clinical depression. If you are experiencing these feelings, speak to a psychiatrist or a trusted family member. Remember, the way to conquer depression is by opening up and talking to someone. Unpacking your feelings and emotions to make sense of it all is a fantastic way to move forward with your recovery and your life.

TESTING

Known as a positive step during the stages of grief, during the testing phase you could still experience hopelessness and depression but begin to see the brighter side of things. You may feel as if the dark cloud is lifting. When you reach this stage, you will begin to look for ways to adapt to your new life with limb loss. Testing is a good place to be mentally and emotionally as you begin to feel positive and the outlook on life begins to not look as dim as when you first lost your limb. The testing stage is a good sign of facing the situation and rising above and getting through the grief of your loss.

BARGAINING

Another common, prominent stage of grief is called bargaining. We have all done this at some point of our lives, yet most don't realize it. Anyone that has endured a traumatic event, such as amputation, usually ends up unknowingly bargaining with themselves. For example, have you ever blamed yourself for everything being your fault? If so, this is a classic case of bargaining. This stage is difficult to overcome because it takes intense thought and soul searching to come to terms with what you are grieving about. Bargaining involves asking questions I label "if only":

- "What if only I had taken better care of myself?"
- "What if only I had been a better person toward my friends?"
- "What if only I had listened to my doctor?"
- "What if only I had taken my medicine?"

You can recognize this stage when you feel the need to place blame on yourself. My good friend, John A., a right-leg below-the-knee amputee, told me, "I blamed myself for not taking my meds and not listening to my doctor." Yet it is human nature to justify what is happening in our lives so, in our emotional state, we plead and make deals to keep from going through this pain. Bargaining is a way to protect ourselves from the painful and harsh reality of limb loss. This is normal, yet do your best to recognize this as bargaining, which could be harmful. If you have these thoughts and questions, seek professional guidance to help you through this stage.

ACCEPTANCE

Acceptance is a stage that is critical to your emotional recovery. After removing yourself from the tough bargaining stage, we can describe the acceptance phase as a reawakening of your life. Acceptance is when you feel positive about the outlook of your life and you have the desire to reengage. Reaching the acceptance stage of your limb loss will promote feelings of being capable of accomplishing anything you set your mind to do. The feelings of gloom should lift, and you will possess newfound freedom. In the acceptance phase, good days outnumber the bad and hope increases, paving a path toward a bright future. The transition from grief, anger, denial, depression, anxiety, and bargaining to acceptance brings forth rich feelings that your life is worth living. Still, reaching acceptance is the hardest stage of grief to attain because of the immense emotional and physical trauma most amputees endure. Keep in mind that the acceptance stage is a true milestone of bravery, a true marker of what you are made of. Acceptance of your limb loss is a giant leap and the beginning of a wonderful transition toward getting the life you once knew back.

COMPULSIVE BEHAVIOR PATTERNS

Amputation is a crisis because everything in your life has changed, and each amputee handles the situation differently. Often, during times of crisis, many react by displaying self-destructive behaviors, attempting to seek "relief" from the deep and hurtful emotions associated with limb loss; these are considered compulsive behaviors. Although everyone is different, these behaviors could become excessive and damaging if left unchecked. Compulsive behaviors can include being a workaholic, and even overachieving. Although they can be perceived as positive attributes, these behaviors can be detrimental to mental health and relationships and cause major suffering.

Drugs and alcohol are associated with codependency, the same as other excessive compulsive behaviors such as overeating, gambling, and binge-watching television. All these factors could damage our underlying mental health and stability. With many amputees experiencing anger, depression, and pain, a high percentage of them trying to cope become addicted to drugs or alcohol. Recovering from addiction is a tough road to maneuver, and many amputees trying to escape addiction have an even bigger challenge in front of them. Why? Amputees attempting to recover from addiction are impeded by critical issues often unforeseen related to their physical or mental disabilities. The rates are shocking. It has been reported that 40 to 50 percent of people with orthopedic disabilities, spinal cord injuries, amputations, or vision impairment can be classified as heavy drinkers or drug users.[4] This means that the substance abuse rates of people with amputations and other disabilities are two to four times higher than people without disabilities.

During the first days after limb loss, pain is treated through drugs to help make you comfortable, and this is when addiction can start. Earlier I discussed different opioids and narcotics that are used during the recovery process. These drugs help manage pain; however, they are highly addictive, and there is the apparent risk with prolonged use of becoming addicted. It is commonly believed that when a doctor prescribes a pill, they expect us to take it. Though you should follow doctors' orders, don't make the mistake of confusing addiction with simply taking a medication because your doctor prescribed it. You must be careful because you can easily fall into the drug addiction trap. Your ongoing treatments will involve seeing more than one physician, each with a unique set of drugs ready to be prescribed for you. Common sense tells us the more drugs, the more significant risk of compulsive addiction. So, either by choice or without awareness, the use of drugs and alcohol could escalate into the danger stages of minor to major dependence.

Unfortunately, many amputees possess addictive personalities, which makes it easy to fall victim to taking drugs long after they have met their medical needs. The problem is that it's difficult to determine whether someone is genuinely experiencing pain or pretending only to receive drug therapy. This is a significant dilemma and a catch-22 because amputees do experience phantom pains and sensations along with physical pain all wrapped into one. These scenarios make it virtually impossible for a doctor to distinguish between actual pain and phantom or imaginary pain.

The recovery success rate for chronic pain patients who are addicted to pain medications is extremely low because of increased tolerance to most pain medications. If you reach a stage where the medicine isn't enough to ease the pain—be careful and responsible. These could be warning signs of early addiction. Pain medication increases could cause quick dependency and reduced chances for a healthy life. Soon, this increase could go from a compulsive obsession to a full-blown drug addiction. Additionally, if you reach this stage, you risk alienating your friends and family and losing their support.

My depression almost got the best of me. It wasn't drugs. Alcohol was my choice because, at first, my limb loss seemed unbearable. My emotions were a tangled mess, and it got so bad that I sadly considered suicide. However, I knew I needed help, so I stopped drinking and sought professional help. I recognized there was too much to live for and considered my wife, kids, parents, siblings, cousins, and grand-children and how it would affect them. I dreaded the idea of leaving a legacy of giving up and taking the simple way out. I thought long and hard about how my death would affect the lives of the ones I love the most. So I stepped up and took on the responsibility of getting well emotionally and physically. My deep love for my family pulled me out of the depths of depression. Throughout my life I have met my share of adversity, yet I was reminded that I've never been known to quit—and losing my leg was no exception. The genuine love I had for everyone around me pushed me into another trajectory and allowed me to nurture the need to take care of others during my survival mode. This revela-tion alone delivered me out of the black hole of depression, which I had fallen into and almost never returned.

Symptoms of depression can lead to hitting rock bottom. Protect yourself and your family from the danger signs of depression. Be aware of them and avoid the path of self-destruction. Chemical dependency kills people physically and emotionally. If you feel you are in trouble, it is vital to seek professional help. Remember, never feel guilty or ashamed about trying to mend your broken self. Feeling broken is nor-mal, and recovery takes perseverance, patience, and, most of all, massive amounts of dedication and heart. The emotional recovery after limb loss is enough of a burden without the added ugliness of substance abuse or other addictive behaviors. These compulsions only further destroy your self-esteem and will bring you down. Remember, life is not over after limb loss. All the good things you deserve will come when you find a healthy balance in all aspects of your life. Work hard, listen, and do everything within your power to maintain that precious balance.

However, experiencing emotional upheavals is unavoidable, espe-cially during the grieving stages after limb loss. It is natural to wonder about where your life is headed and what role you will play moving forward. Everything, at first, will seem out of control and difficult to see beyond your immediate circumstances. You may experience the lowest of lows, making it seemingly impossible to get your life back. Lift the burdens and lighten your emotional load by talking to family or friends about how you feel. Being open about your feelings is a positive step toward living the best life possible.

I once visited Thomas J., an amputee friend, in the hospital. He said, "When I was at my lowest point with my depression, I fought ruthlessly to remain independent. I wanted to be self-sufficient." Thomas also told me he had fought hard, and even wore himself out, trying to do everything that he normally did before he lost his legs, but he never sought help. After hearing Thomas's story, I realized the importance of asking for help from others. Don't feel guilty asking for help. My limb loss placed the burden on my wife left me with immense guilt. It was difficult to see everything falling in her lap: finances, household chores, taking care of me. Watching her struggle getting me to and from the doctor and in and out of my wheelchair saddened me. Together with this guilt I felt unworthy and avoided the ugly reality that I couldn't do certain things. Eventually, I knew I had to ask for help and came to terms with it.

To reach this discovery yourself, you must allow for quiet time to reflect and experience the depth of your feelings. There isn't any shame in embracing your emotions and taking the time in accepting the reality of your situation. Being able to feel what is happening around you is crucial to living and being in the moment. Early in life most of us are taught to ignore feelings of sadness, hurt, and confusion. Experiencing severe physical trauma pushes us to completely disconnect from our feelings in an act of avoidance. We want to run away, which derives from our natural instinct to survive. However, prolonging this mode could render you unable to reconnect with the world around you once again. Reconnecting involves opening up and accepting your feelings, good and bad, and acknowledging the need to heal yourself. This may seem easy, but it's extremely hard to do because every one of us is afraid of losing ourselves and admitting something is wrong. Yet our primal human instinct is to avoid bad feelings at all costs and numb ourselves by turning inward, avoiding what is uncomfortable instead of enduring the pain.

Turning inward is healthy, to a point. Still, don't look inward and stay there by ignoring the pain, feelings, and everyone around you. Emotionally, this is a disastrous place to be. Avoid allowing yourself to be closed off, and embrace what you are feeling so you can achieve real recovery. For a brief time I turned off my feelings and didn't want to talk to anyone. In my mind it was impossible to humble myself to the emotional or physical support from anyone. It made me feel weak and helpless. The last thing I wanted was to be a burden to everyone around me. I felt inadequate, and the word "freak" even entered my mind a time or two. However, it wasn't long before I recognized that I had to accept the fact that I couldn't do everything I used to do. Routine tasks that once were second nature now took extra time and my full concentration to complete. My world took on a different shape and everything required more time, strength, concentration—and help—to accomplish.

It is perfectly normal to allow yourself a brief period of emotional self-indulgence. Discovering what you are capable of is a level of personal growth that many people are never fortunate enough to experience. Throughout your recovery you may surprise yourself with a brand-new level of awareness and spiritual reconnection. Finding peace within comes from opening up, taking the time, and sitting quietly with your thoughts. Acceptance of what you feel is crucial to moving forward. Lifting yourself up emotionally can be uncomfortable, but overall, it's an ongoing process that needs to be accepted as an integral part of your life.

Remember, your family and friends are going through this recovery alongside you. Keep yourself in check and treat others around you with respect and kindness. Do your best to not project anger or frustration toward others. These are the people who love you, and no matter what you are feeling, make sure they know how much you appreciate their help. Depression can alter your rational mind and make you act out uncontrollably and possibly do things you may regret. Ultimately, you need these people in your corner to help you get back to living your life. When you treat someone with disrespect or show anger toward them, it pushes them away, which only hurts you. I've learned this the hard way. One evening I yelled at my wife and snapped at her terribly. I felt enraged and out of control. The moment I screamed, I saw she was hurt and confused. My heart sank as I realized how much she had sacrificed by waiting on me hand and foot and helping me every step of the way. From that moment I knew I had to treat her with respect and keep my temper and outbursts at bay or I would push her away—for good. I still struggle in this area, and I've sought a professional counselor to work hard and fix this about myself.

Although despite strong efforts the intense struggle of being an amputee can take its toll. You are human, but do your absolute best to monitor your reactions toward other people. Do not belittle or make them feel unwanted. This makes the other person believe they are useless to you, and that is an empty place to be in. Have you ever felt you were useless to someone? It doesn't feel good. Feeling useless is not a good feeling, is it? Try your best, no matter what you are going through, to not make that same mistake with others. Being kind, patient, and understanding with everyone around during this troublesome time is an essential part of a healthy recovery.

Richard Bach, author of *Illusions: The Adventures of a Reluctant Messiah* (1989), wrote, "What the caterpillar calls the end of the world, the master calls a butterfly."[5] Emerging back into your life and returning to doing what you love, depending on your limb loss, maybe prove to be simple or extremely difficult. The reality is there may be activities you used to do that, unfortunately, are almost impossible to return to. Remember, this is not the end of the world. If you can't enjoy a sport or activity, there is nothing wrong with being a spectator and being around fans and friends. There isn't any shame here. When this happens, explore other activities or sports you may enjoy. However, if attending an event as a spectator stirs up painful emotions, that is okay, too. As you adjust to your new life, you will develop new interests in different sports and activities. Today, technology offers many options to choose from that allow amputees of almost all different limb amputations to pick up the pieces and get back to doing what they love. After my amputation, never did I imagine that I would end up writing books for a living. Yet my limb loss sent my life into a totally new trajectory. This new career is a daily reminder of the beauty of adapting to change. It doesn't replace the loss, but being open-minded and willing to look at other interests can open the door to endless possibilities.

HOW TO HELP YOUR DEPRESSION AND GRIEF

Depression is a serious issue and should never be taken lightly. I have discovered that there are many things you can try to lift yourself up, stay positive, and overcome limb loss depression.

Sleep and Rest

Getting enough rest allows your body and mind to recuperate and re-generate. I know that sleep and depression are a double-edged sword. Depression can cause sleep problems and sleep problems can lead to having depression. Most symptoms of depression make themselves present before the onset of sleep problems. Yet, unfortunately, some sleep disorders can occur before signs of depression set in. If you are experiencing sleep problems after your limb loss, seek help from a sleep professional. There are specialists who can assist you in figuring out the barriers to getting a good night's rest. If the sleep problem escalates and continues, reach out and seek medical help. Doctors, along with sleep study professionals, should be able to determine the root causes to help in getting better sleep for your overall health and well-being.

Getting Out and Being Active

Getting out of the house and doing daily activities are excellent avenues to fight depression. My amputee friend Gloria W., a right-arm ampu-tee, told me that when she goes to the grocery store, she takes her time shopping. "I enjoy being out," she said. "Makes me feel normal again." Depending on your limb loss, try your best not to let your amputation stop you from getting out and enjoying life. Getting back to doing things you did before the limb loss is highly recommended and fun. Being active and doing what you love is essential to your recovery and mental health. Being around friends and going to events you enjoy are excellent ways to beat depression. Allowing yourself the freedom to be in the moment will help you overcome depression in more ways than you will expect.

· *10* ·

Friendships, Family, and Children

As we express our gratitude, we must never forget that the highest appreciation is not to utter words, but to live by them.

—John F. Kennedy

IMMEDIATE FAMILY

It didn't take long after my limb loss to recognize the importance of family and friends providing care and caregiver support. The goal of this book is to help every amputee get back the life they once knew, and the same wish is for their family who help and support behind the scenes. Your family and friends are essential to your recovery, and loved ones are often overlooked and never recognized. There is an ever-present need to support the caregivers of limb loss patients because your family is human, too. While standing beside you, each one is experiencing their own limb loss journey in tandem with you. Being a family caregiver, just like an amputee, you probably have a million questions to what is happening around you. Perhaps you are confused, frustrated, sad, and even worried about the effects of the limb loss on your life. Wherever you find yourself and whatever the role you play in your loved one's life, whether a close friend, family member, spouse, or child, never forget you are instrumental in helping your loved one every step of the way. Most family caregivers, through the trauma and excitement, are underappreciated, and my goal is to shed light on those who are needed the most. I know how important this subject is after seeing firsthand what my wife went through: the struggle, the pain, the hurt alongside me. I am going to address those most affected by this critical situation: the amputee and caregiver. As a new amputee you may have family, friends, and even children involved in your recovery. And as a family member, friend, or child, you may have found yourself unexpectedly thrown into the role of caregiver. I am going to shed much needed light from both sides:

- Caregiver to amputee
- Amputee to caregiver

If you are reading this and seeking answers as the caregiver, I will provide a firsthand glimpse into what an amputee experiences to help you understand better from the amputee's perspective. I believe that having perspectives from both sides is vital for a healthy and strong recovery for everyone involved. Perhaps you have a loved one getting ready to go through amputation or maybe you've had someone who has just lost their limb. The intent is to help define firsthand what you will be dealing with. The information gleaned should provide direct insight into precisely what your loved one is experiencing. Understanding this information should help you cope, manage, and deliver the best care for your loved one.

FAMILY AND RELATIONSHIPS
AFTER AMPUTATION: CAREGIVER'S VIEW

Studies and reports have shown that more relationships end in divorce because of poor communication and misunderstandings. During a crisis, such as amputation, human nature reverts to the primal instinct to protect ourselves through distancing and withdrawal from anything that causes pain. Limb loss is devastating, and even talking about your partner's amputation, at this critical stage, could be painful and cause confusion, resentment, and frustration. These feelings could lead to relationship disaster. Even the strongest relationships could be tested when both people are subjected to weathering a traumatic event such as amputation. Remember to be strong and levelheaded because a crisis of this nature could make you feel like throwing in the towel.

The days leading up to my amputation, my wife and I were both confused and scared about where our lives were headed. For both of us the feelings of despair were overpowering, causing massive stress and frustration. I felt washed up as I now had a front row seat watching her suffer by being cast into the role of primary caregiver, working to keep our household together. I wanted to help her as much as I could, but I was powerless, helpless, and vulnerable. To add to our stress, before the limb loss we had been going through some of the hardest times of our lives. Our relationship was critically strained from my recent job loss and other significant financial worries. Yet we stood together through it all and, without doubt, going through the experience of limb loss together, figuring out what and what not to do brought us even closer. What we endured together made our relationship and marriage stronger.

Still, my wife worried about everything in our lives and where we were headed. I could see the strain, pressure, and all-out worry about our finances and the burden of taking care of me on her face. I could see her straining to keep up the hectic pace with doctor appointments, errands for medicine, and the pressure of working to pay the bills. They were taking their toll. The financial strain was intense and, from my perspective, it was rough, and it made me feel horrible inside, even guilty and helpless. I realized that the only way to help her was to get tough and fight for my life. The saving grace was that she and I talked through the situation and worked together on what we had to do. Each of us remained open and honest about our primary fears and concerns. Strong communication and a willingness to embrace the situation allowed us both to heal and move forward, and I believe we would not have made it otherwise.

Perhaps you may feel this way and are concerned about how the limb loss is affecting your life. This is a natural response because everything, from this point forward, will take on a different aspect. Essentially, your loved one's limb loss will have a dramatic impact on your life, yet the goal is to be patient and allow understanding and compassion to remain. Over time, most families learn to cope and come to terms with the situation. Understand there will be obstacles, difficulties, major challenges, and bumps in the road all aimed to deter and discourage. Be aware of this and do your best to address them positively and not to let them get you down. Having doubt and fear naturally makes you wonder how life will be in the future. There is apprehension and a strong urgency for answers on what you don't understand because we are human and feeling this way is natural. As you move along the recovery journey, expect major questions, concerns, and doubts about taking care of your loved one and living your life. The best way to address the situation is to understand that your loved one is experiencing one of the hardest events of their life and needs unfiltered support and care. Remember, you must do your best to place the needs of your loved one over yours to provide optimal care. Being there 100 percent is vital to their recovery. This advice may sound a touch self-centered, but the care needed after amputation is unmatched and they will need your undivided attention.

Sarah W., the wife of my right-leg amputee friend, Todd W., was scared about her husband's limb loss. "I didn't know what to do or who to talk to," she said. "But I finally got up the courage and started asking nurses and doctors what to do." Once she talked to the doctors, she received sound advice on the care of her husband. "I felt better and less confused," she told me after speaking with the doctor. As the primary caregiver, it will be a challenge for you in sorting out what is needed, but remember, you have an essential role in the healing journey of your loved one.

Clearly, limb loss is an emotionally charged, traumatic event for everyone. When you are facing stepping into the caregiver role, it may be even harder to witness the hurt alongside your loved one. The nature of the situation and feeling helpless could be emotionally draining on you. With the varying degree of high emotions as a caregiver, it is natural to experience your own emotional pain. No one wants to see a loved one hurt, and it may affect you, so stay strong and be there as much as you can. Experiencing these emotions with your loved one could overwhelm and make you feel like shutting down, which is a natural reflex response. The key to overcoming this is to communicate how you feel and show your compassion for the situation. Open up, be considerate, be willing and practical to provide the best care for your loved one. Caring for a loved one with limb loss takes understanding, knowledge, skill, and, most of all, love. However, even with all of this in mind, it is difficult to know where to begin.

One of the best suggestions for you as a family caregiver to help in making this a smoother transition is to speak to your loved ones and ask about their immediate concerns or about any urgent needs. Understanding their immediate needs and concerns will get things started on the right track. Your loved one will find comfort in knowing that you are concerned about their immediate needs and will listen. Recovery is a team effort, and throughout the recovery process, it doesn't take long to realize how much they need you. Remember, they need your support no matter how they react, and your goal is to be strong and persevere, leading through example. Amputees have enough to worry about, so recognizing their immediate needs is an excellent way of providing support and encouragement. Every little bit of help and support from you aids in the long road to recovery.

TALKING TO OTHER AMPUTEES

A great way to learn is by example and by talking to amputees. Set up meetings with other amputees to discuss helpful ideas and tips in making recovery smoother. If you do not know any immediate amputees, reach out to organizations such as The Amputee Coalition's Certified Peer Visitor program (www.amputee-coalition.org). Understanding what to expect on the road to recovery can help you every step of the way.

FAMILY AND RELATIONSHIPS
AFTER AMPUTATION: AMPUTEE'S VIEW

Early in your recovery, you may find yourself immediately surrounded by family, your spouse, close friends, even children who are willing and ready to step in and help take care of you. Never forget these people are there to give the best of themselves—for you. Help them help you by taking the guesswork out of your care by telling them what you need. Open up and let them know your expectations because the more they know, the better they can help. Let them know about any emotions, discomfort, or pain you're experiencing, which allows for a long-term, positive outcome effects in building a trusting and supportive relationship. Remember, during your recovery you need all the support you can get, and this is not the time to tear down people around you. Lift them up and let them help you.

ACCEPTANCE OR
REJECTION BY FRIENDS AND FAMILY

J. K. Rowling, author of *Harry Potter and the Goblet of Fire*, once said, "Understanding is the first step to acceptance, and only with acceptance can there be recovery."[1]

Most amputees deal with acceptance or rejection from friends and family. I was no exception. Right after my amputation there was a barrage of people around me. Each person showed concern, and many volunteered to help me and my family through the crisis. However, over time, there was a slow fade of interest and they disappeared from my life. One by one, phone calls ceased, visits stopped, and even encouraging text messages ground to a jarring halt. At first I had struggled with this. I felt lost, rejected, and undone. I blamed myself for their absence, believing that there was something wrong with me worse than my limb loss.

I became angry and asked, "Why!!? What was wrong with me?" I couldn't believe they turned their back on me. I was disheartened and in total disbelief because I thought I knew these people, yet their absence told me the real story—I didn't know them at all. I was the same person with the same talents, dreams, ideas, and beliefs. The only thing that had changed was my leg. So in my mind there had to be something else.

I was wrong.

The truth is some people simply cannot handle your limb loss and the stress or change it creates in their lives. Over time most friends and family members come to grips with your situation and adapt. Unfortunately, people will come and go from your life, so do your best to understand. What you're going through is hard on them emotionally. So if they distance themselves, remember it is not you. Whether they accept or reject you and your limb loss is their "baggage," so do not take on the burden that you as a person are to blame. There are some people who need extra time to process your situation and, in most instances, this slight rejection comes from a good heart, a place of love, and genuine concern for your welfare. They just don't want to see you hurting and it pains them to see you suffer. Still, some people can handle and internalize it rather quickly. Others wish to not see you in pain and decide to flee from what hurts them.

Life gets better when you come to terms with others not accepting you. You only have yourself, and it will take strength and determination to transition into your new life. The key is to remain focused and undeterred and to not to let people skew your outlook. Remain open by allowing people to come into your life and remain steadfast in not blaming those who leave. People will walk out of your life for reasons only they know. Remember, it may be because it's hard for them to accept your limb loss and simply can't comprehend what you're going through. Some feel uncomfortable and don't know what to say when they are around you. These are all normal human reactions that should be expected.

Friends are one thing, but when family members can't resolve their feelings about your limb loss it can be extremely hard. Being without some of your closer family members is hurtful. The fact is you cannot control how people will react or respond to your limb loss, no matter who they are. If someone in your family can't accept your loss, be patient and give them space. Adjusting to your new life is an arduous enough task without the added pressure of getting people to accept the new you. This is solely their responsibility, and you must understand, even though it may be difficult, the burden is on them and not you. However, losing friends and family may create a massive void in your life, but having patience and compassion toward them can help mend the heart and relationships. Over time you will discover there will be many people willing to be a part of your life. There is freedom and peace in knowing that people will leave, and that others will remain and thrive by helping you recover.

RELATIONSHIPS WITH CHILDREN AFTER AMPUTATION: AMPUTEE'S VIEW

Children are special, but some may not cope well with your limb loss, especially small children who may not understand what has happened. They may see you as broken, or that something is wrong, making them feel scared. If this happens do not be hurt by their reactions. Children are amazingly sensitive and aware of the world around them. The way a child's mind works may make them feel responsible for your limb loss; it's easy for a child to misinterpret your amputation and blame themselves for your misfortune. I once spoke to an eleven-year-old girl, Tonya H. Her dad had just lost both his legs in an automobile crash. The accident happened after her father and mother had gotten into an argument. The father stormed out and jumped in the car. Just before he pulled away, Tonya had begged him not to go. He didn't listen. Ten minutes later he was involved in the crash that took his two legs and almost killed him. Tonya, being a child, felt responsible for her dad's leg loss. "It's my fault he will never walk again!" she cried. I explained there wasn't anything she did or could have done that would have prevented this accident, yet she took on massive guilt as if it were all her fault.

Give your children the chance to talk about their feelings. Let them know it is okay to say how they feel. Tell them your genuine feelings, assure them you are healing, and explain that it will take time for everyone to adjust to your recovery. Young children cannot grasp the reality of what is happening, so reassure them you are still who you are. Comfort them as normal by doing your best to be involved in their lives. Read bedtime stories or bake their favorite cookie; whatever it is, do your best to show normalcy. Explain that things may be different, but you intend to be there, 100 percent. Most of all, let them know your limb loss not their fault.

In times of crisis some children express their fears with anger or aggressiveness. Other children may withdraw themselves from you emotionally and physically. Be patient because emotionally, just like you and me, a child needs to process the changes around them. Children must be allowed time to adjust to your limb loss, plus your new image. Do not be hurt or take it personally if your child does not open up to you or shies away at first. Allow your child to react in their own way, and give them space. Some older children may feel more comfortable talking to someone else or a close friend instead of confiding in you. That's okay. Let them. Don't push them to talk to you right away. Forcing conversations when they are not ready can only push them further away, and you will then run the risk of your child distancing and withdrawing from you further for a longer period of time. Do your best to be understanding and patient, reassuring them that they can take all the time they need to process what is happening. Let them know you understand and most of all, allow them space to grieve and come to terms with your limb loss in their lives. Over time healing will begin and your relationship with your kids will be the best it has ever been. Have faith in that.

INFANT AND CHILD AMPUTEES: COPING WITH LIMB LOSS

Every day babies are born across the globe with congenital amputations and limb deficiencies. One in every two thousand babies born has a congenital amputation or limb deficiency comprising absent extremities such as hands, fingers, toes, or whole limbs. Being born or growing up as an amputee child is immensely challenging. Today's youth have to deal with the pressures of school, social media, and society. For a teenager the negative aspect of missing a limb or how they look can be almost impossible to manage. Young women amputees have an even more difficult road because of puberty, hormones, and coming of age all mixed with the feelings of inadequacy from a missing limb. All of this can take its toll and be devastating. As a parent do everything in your power to be understanding and compassionate and listen to your children. Be open and reassure them they can always talk to you. For the best advice ask other amputee parents for tips on providing the best environment for your child.

RECOVERY: MOVING ON WITH YOUR LIFE

As you navigate through recovery the day will come where you must start thinking about rebuilding your life. Steps need to be taken to embrace an alternative way to live with your limb loss. Your life has a new purpose, and soon you will find a major reset leading you to discover a new meaning and direction for your life that includes building relationships with family and friends as you emerge through recovery. Welcoming lost family back into your life is essential, and do your best to allow them to experience your newfound life with you. Remember, getting back to relationships, understanding people's roles, intentions, while accepting the loss and gain of family and friends and even children is essential to your overall recovery.

· 11 ·

Relationships and Sexuality

For a marriage relationship to flourish, there must be intimacy. It takes an enormous amount of courage to say to your spouse, "This is me. I'm not proud of it—in fact, I'm a little embarrassed by it—but this is who I am."

—Bill Hybels

GETTING BACK TO SEXUALITY

A few weeks after my surgery I sat alone looking at myself in the mirror. It was hard to see myself, my leg missing, vulnerable and forever changed. My reflection showed more than I wanted because I saw a man that was broken, incomplete, even empty. Instantly, I felt embarrassed and worried about how my wife would react to seeing me this way. My mind raced with questions. Would my stump gross her out? Would she still be attracted to me sexually? How could I make love to her this way? These were hard questions I had to face, and the beginning of my understanding that my sexual relationship was about to undergo a significant change.

Talking about sexuality as an amputee is, at first, an extremely sensitive and private subject. Even though the importance of understanding sexuality as an amputee should be at the forefront, there isn't much discussion or emphasis about sexual intimacy available for amputees. Sex is important to everyone's life and relationships, and I believe we need to address the subject head-on by breaking it down into the most pertinent topics that many are reluctant to talk about.

115

For amputees there are deep-rooted concerns that become apparent, such as rejection, acceptance, and the fear of limited physical ability to perform sexually. However, with most amputations, especially lower, it is recommended to wait six to eight weeks before returning to sexual intimacy. Not only is the waiting period designed to allow you to heal, but it also gives you time to prepare yourself mentally and physically for intimacy. Intimacy and sexuality are personal and private, and everyone has different expectations on what they need and want. Some amputees may be eager and ready before six weeks, and for others six weeks is way too soon, especially if you're still experiencing pain and discomfort. Plus, you may experience a slower recovery period, which can make you feel less sexual desire. Either way, these are common situations and there isn't anything wrong with you. You are human, and when there is pain involved, it can prove challenging to think of sex or pleasure in anything other than what you are experiencing. Additionally, pain medications and other medicines could contribute to you having less desire to reengage in sexual activity. As humans, we condition our brains to "flee" from anything that hurts. It only makes sense not to want to engage in sexual activity because of the physical pain along with the severe emotional trauma associated with limb loss. Sexual desire and the urge to partake in intimacy often disappear after this form of trauma. However, the good news is that the desire to reengage will return. Therefore, it is imperative that you give yourself permission to take your time. Be patient because not feeling the desire for sex is temporary; if it takes longer for your desire to return, it is natural to feel as if something is wrong with you. It may discourage you as you feel your desire will never come back. Hang in there and be patient, because as you heal emotionally and physically, your sexual desire will return.

However, as with anything in life, when you don't do something for a while it may take time to get back into the swing of things. Sexual intimacy and ability aren't any different. Being intimate for the first time after amputation may seem awkward and even frightening. You may feel out of sorts, as if you forgot what to do or how to engage. Think of getting back into a sexual relationship and intimacy just like riding a bicycle. No matter how long it has been since you rode a bike, once you hop on it all seems to come back to you. However, depending on your specific limb loss, you may need to relearn different ways to perform sexually with your partner. What used to be normal and comfortable could now be a significant issue. Everything from position, strength, stamina, and even taking off your clothes for the first time can be emotionally difficult. There are emotions and deep-rooted feelings that could be amplified, such as feeling embarrassed or intimidated of being naked in front of your partner for the first time. If prolonged, these emotions could become problematic and ultra-traumatic, with the fear growing into worry of spousal rejection and vulnerability of being on "exhibit." Sexual intimacy involves many things, and the simple act of undressing in front of your partner may be traumatic and emotionally draining.

Peggy Chenoweth, a below-the-knee amputee and mother of two, wrote,

> It took nearly six months post-amputation until I was ready for intimacy. This extended time was due to an infection in my stump, but in retrospect, it was also because I was feeling ugly. I simply wasn't eager to be seen. For partners of an amputee, patience is imperative! I was desperate for reassurance that I was attractive, and that I was still viewed as a whole woman. My body shape had drastically changed, and it took a while to learn and to accept how I looked and felt.[11]

For me, sexual intimacy is a subject close to home, and it has taken me quite a while to feel comfortable being intimate with my wife. It was rough going because at first, she thought I was not attracted to her. That was not the case, yet I had difficulty making her understand that it wasn't her. She was afraid that I didn't find her desirable, yet it was the other way around. I was petrified that she was not sexually attracted to me any longer. This worry made me feel closed off about sex because I was too afraid to find out. I wanted to make love to her and had desire, but I wanted to hide because of my mental image of myself. Sex was a massive wall I couldn't seem to get over. I would look at myself, my stump, and my body as a whole and could not see myself in the same way. I felt broken, unmasculine, vulnerable, and unattractive. My major mistake was I assumed my wife saw me in the same way.

I was wrong because she didn't.

Admittedly, I remained self-conscious in the bedroom setting and worried about how I looked without clothes on. Even though I know now, my wife sees me as the same man, I still perceive myself as startling and incomplete, even though I know both those things are not valid or even true. Yet with lovemaking, the struggle is real. I still feel vulnerable and unattractive in the bedroom but over time things have gotten better.

Maybe you are experiencing these same feelings. If so, this is normal. I have an excellent amputee friend, Jerry M., who lost both of his legs below the knee to a traumatic fall. Jerry opened up and confided in me. He said he didn't want his wife to see him without his prostheses on, so he wore it all the time. He even wore them while he slept for fear of his wife seeing his legs in the morning.

Feeling vulnerable and fearful is hard to admit for most of us. Society tells us that men need to be tough, strong, and masculine. They must perform like stallions in the bedroom. And women must be supersexy. Society also states that if either doesn't live up to these false expectations, there must be something wrong.

This is simply not true.

Remember, you haven't changed other than your physical appearance. You are still you and the person your partner cares about. No matter your amputation, there isn't anything wrong with you, so be brave and do your best to express your feelings and concerns about intimacy with your partner. Being open about how you feel will strengthen your bond and help your partner understand what you're feeling and what is happening. During this time in your life, this is a critical element in strengthening your relationship.

In feeling attractive and masculine, most male amputees can get away with hiding their limb loss. With a lower limb amputation, a man can wear pants that make it difficult to see their missing limb. Women, on the other hand, have a troublesome time hiding limb loss. Every woman desires to be wanted and strives to be beautiful in their own way, yet limb loss makes most women feel less sexy, inadequate, and even embarrassed in an intimate setting. Many women, throughout their normal lives, like to wear dresses, lingerie, and even sexy shorts and undergarments, which leave little room in disguising any type of limb loss. When an amputee woman experiences fear and deep bouts of anxiety about showing themselves, it could have a drastic effect on their mental and emotional state.

Men and women are completely different with attractiveness, sex, and intimacy. Most men don't worry as much about their physical appearance as much as women, yet in the bedroom setting, most men and women worry about their outward appearance and how they're seen sexually. Every woman wants to look sexy and suitable for their partner, but in being an amputee, this can be a fear-filled event with how their partner sees them in the bedroom. These fears could become troublesome, making a person want to avoid sex.

Sex is vital to a healthy partnership. Avoiding sexual intimacy can put an immense strain on any relationship and could also make your partner feel unwanted or undesired. Once this happens, there is a major risk of resentment and ill feelings, which could lead to significant relationship issues. Remember, make sure you do not use your amputation as a "crutch" to mask avoidance of sex and intimacy. Take your time to heal, but do not ignore your relationship because it could place what you hold dear in jeopardy. The struggle can be substantial when you have a partner who wishes to be sexually active and you do not. Be open and talk to your partner about your feelings and issues. Ask them to be patient and understanding about your internal conflict. Open communication will aid in creating a deeper and more meaningful relationship between you both. Often, you may be incorrect to think that your partner sees you negatively. However, more often than not, they love you and only see who you are on the inside—not what you look like on the outside. Yet be patient, as it may be difficult for your partner at the onset. Do your best to be understanding and keep the channels of communication always open. Invite them to voice their genuine concerns about your limb loss and keep working together to find alternative ways that work for both of you.

No matter how long it takes for you to get back the desire to be intimate, never neglect your partner. Remain loving and caring by touching, hugging, cuddling, and kissing them. Offer intimate body massages and remain attentive by showing that closeness and intimacy that don't have to result in sex. Through compassion, patience, understanding, love, and other intimate alternatives, you and your partner will eventually break down all physical and emotional barriers your limb loss may have built. Show your partner you still care by going the extra mile through gestures of care and kindness. Respect your partner's feelings, and through positive actions affirm that you desire to reestablish a healthy sexual relationship when you're ready.

When you feel you are ready for sexual intimacy, depending on your specific limb loss, you may discover or have trouble in performing various sexual positions. There isn't anything wrong with you if this happens. Remember, things have only changed physically, so now put your creativity to work in finding fresh ways that work. Talk to your partner and work out alternative ways and explore the options. Take this opportunity to even spice things up by trying new things you never had before. Approach this with an open mind in finding new ways to have fun with sex. The adventurous approach releases tension and reduces the stress by emphasizing the fun part, taking the focus off your limb loss.

DATING AFTER AMPUTATION

I talked to my amputee friend George W., whose wife left him after his amputation. He was terrified of being alone because he felt disgusting and undesirable. He thought no one would ever love him again. George's self-image had reached rock bottom. He worried about how he would ever meet someone new with his disability.

George's concern was genuine, yet Aimee Mullins, actress, successful model, and double-leg amputee said in an interview with the *Huffington Post,* "People presume my disability has to do with being an amputee, but that's not the case; our insecurities are our disabilities, and I struggle with those as does everyone."[22] Aimee's quote reveals a strong point. Limb loss is a disability, but who you are as a person truly counts. Insecurities can be even more debilitating than limb loss. It can be complicated for some of us who are single to re-establish our lives and build new relationships. There is genuine fear in starting new relationships and opening up sexually in a new relationship after limb loss. Most of us, before limb loss, are comfortable getting undressed and being sexually intimate, but now things have changed. If you are single, you will meet someone new and the first encounter of being naked can be tricky, even frightening. There also other factors besides your limb loss, such as body image, weight, physical health, plus everyday human imperfections that make it difficult when meeting someone new. So in new intimate situations, be yourself and relax. Do not concentrate on your imperfections, especially your limb loss. Take the focus elsewhere by displaying your outstanding traits and who you genuinely are because honesty and heart will win every time. Even though it may be hard at first when meeting someone new, be open and forthcoming about your limb loss and allow them to process it in their own way.

At first the world of dating may be extremely awkward as an amputee. Society promotes for people to not discriminate against anyone with disabilities or physical challenges, and still there are some people who do. However, just because someone isn't attracted to you doesn't mean it's because of your limb loss. Everyone has different tastes. It can be as simple as someone being attracted to blondes or a certain build or stature. These are factors beyond your control, so never automatically assume someone isn't interested in you because of your appearance. Do your best to believe a new relationship can thrive because of your amputation. The laws of attraction are unexplained and remain a mystery on what exactly brings people together. What repels someone from being with you may just be the magnet that attracts the love of your life. Despite your limb loss, personality, traits, and personal preferences play a significant role in any new relationship.

Being upfront about your limb loss is vitally important at the onset of any new relationship. Use your best judgment on when the time is right to discuss it, but allow the other person to get to know you first. Today, some experts believe there is an obvious risk in telling someone upfront about your limb loss. There is fear that they may not be able to handle the situation. Many feel this leaves an amputee open for disappointment and rejection. Of course, with any relationship, there is a significant risk of rejection, but limb loss magnifies it. There are other experts who think it best to establish a relationship first before revealing your limb loss situation if possible. Decide for yourself what you are most comfortable with when approaching a new relationship, but either way the risk of being rejected remains.

Relationships as an amputee are a trial-and-error process and aren't much different from anyone else's. Finding the right someone takes time, so be patient and don't settle for the first person who comes along. In any relationship, whether friendships, dating, or marriage, always make yourself happy and do not settle for less. Recognize that you are uniquely you and deserve only the best, considerate, and most compassionate people in your life. People will come and go, but you are worthy of having the right someone who can appreciate the hardship you have endured. You deserve someone who sees the real person you are on the inside and values who you truly are.

Last, sexuality and relationships include friendships with people of both sexes. Both male and female friends can provide much needed support through your limb loss journey. Nurture these friendships, give back, and do your best to never forget them. New friendships and relationships should be cherished so remember to invest time in them. Pursue the life you desire by being patient in returning to healthy sexual relationships and intimacy when you are ready. Allow yourself to heal, open up, and enjoy closeness with your partner because your enjoyment, giving, and love should last a lifetime.

V

REGAINING YOUR INDEPENDENCE AND LIFE

Independence, Mobility, and Prosthetics

When one door of happiness closes, another opens, but often we look so long at the closed door that we do not see the one that has been opened for us.

—Helen Keller

$\mathcal{B}$eing physically independent as a new amputee should be an essential part of your recovery goals. Whether you are an upper or lower amputee, gaining your independence is one of the first steps in mapping out your life. One way to get there is to accept the use of assistive devices and prosthetics. Sarah J., a left-arm below-the-elbow amputee, told me, "In my experience, there isn't anything I can't do now that I couldn't do before with my prosthetic. I only had to figure out ways to do it differently." One of the most significant aspects of being an amputee is the use of prosthetics and the acceptance of a prosthesis in your life. Initially, a prosthesis may look and feel strange, but once you start using it, the benefits and your perception of it should substantially change. A prosthetic allows freedom, with newfound mobility. It allows you to forego the use of a wheelchair and other assistive devices. Even though both prosthetics and assistive devices play integral roles in gaining back independence, the key is accepting both as fundamental in getting back your life.

Found in *Inspiring Quotes*, Jim Abbott, a professional baseball player born without a right hand, said, "There are millions of people out there ignoring disabilities and accomplishing incredible feats. I learned you could learn to do things differently but do them just as well. I've learned that it's not the disability that defines you, it's how you deal with the challenges the disability presents you with. And I've learned that we have an obligation to the abilities we DO have, not the disability."[11]

There are different assistive devices specifically designed for upper limb amputees that provide the best quality of life. However, many upper limb amputees may or may not need a prosthetic or even choose not to use one. Sarah N., a left-arm below-the-elbow amputee, told me during a peer visit phone call, "I will not fool with a prosthetic. I think I am going to learn how to make the best of my life without one and figure things out on my own." For upper limb amputees who want to use assistive devices, there are many innovations to help them, such as:

- One-Handed Belt
- Easy Open Jar Openers
- One-Handed Cutting Boards
- One-Handed Toothpaste Dispensers
- One-Handed Book Page Holders
- One-Handed Bra Fastener Devices
- One-Handed Bottle Openers
- Hands-Free Dog Leashes

Any one of these devices can help you do everyday tasks and maintain a normal life. Yet the hardest aspect for any upper limb amputee is figuring out ways to do tasks that were once considered routine. At first these tasks may seem impossible, yet human nature almost always prevails. By using your ingenuity and creativity, you can quickly figure out ways to do things around your home and in your life. Reaching this stage in your amputee life is empowering. You will gain much-needed confidence being able to maneuver and perform different tasks with ease.

Whether you have had a hand, arm, or even a finger amputated, you first need to decide if you intend to use a prosthesis or forgo having one. However, with many upper extremity amputations, it may be unnecessary to use a prosthesis. For many upper limb amputees, it is a preference not a necessity, compared to the importance of a prosthesis for lower limb amputees. Many upper limb amputees choose what they call a "passive prosthesis," which is worn predominantly for visual and cosmetic purposes and does not serve in any functional capacity. These kinds of prosthetics help to ease insecurities and make it easier to be seen by others. However, other upper limb amputees choose to use a "functional prosthesis." These prosthetic devices enable you to perform daily tasks along with being worn for visual and cosmetic purposes. A functional prosthesis makes your amputation visually appealing while giving you freedom, functionality, and a profound sense of independence. These prostheses provide useful ways to grip, hold, touch, and even lift objects. Today, technology is vastly improved in the upper prosthetic innovation field. Advancements in prosthetics have delivered new devices that provide practical use through either electric and or body power. Various body-powered prosthetics maneuver with specifically designed harnesses and cable systems that move when the patient moves. Movements such as opening and closing a prosthetic hand for gripping is achieved by the patient's own body movement and strength. The operation of this prosthesis is a simple braking system like that found on a common bicycle. When used, most amputees say they can "feel" the action and the "grip." Companies such as Hanger and Össur are making great technological advances to help almost every upper limb amputee. Research the different choices available based upon your specific needs and decide if you want to use a prosthesis. Discuss with your prosthetist and doctor the options that best fit your lifestyle. Remember, the choice is entirely up to you.

LOWER LIMB MOBILITY WITH ASSISTIVE DEVICES (PREPROSTHETIC)

Using a prosthetic is a necessity for lower limb amputees to get mobile once again. Before having a prosthetic, you will need other assistive devices to move around as they will help with the physical preparation for a prosthetic later in your recovery. Learning to stand, walk, move, and balance will be easier with these assistive devices as you work through your recovery toward a prosthetic.

There are many useful and prominent assistive devices you will encounter, such as:

- Crutches
- Hand crutches

- Canes
- Walkers
- Wheelchairs
- Electric carts

Assistive devices make getting around and performing daily tasks easier. By using assistive devices, you will build strength and reduce strain on other parts of your body. You will undergo different stages of recovery, and specific assistive devices will promote progress and a positive healing process. Speak to your physical therapist, doctor, or prosthetist on the specific equipment you need for your specific situation. These trained professionals should instruct you to use the equipment properly for the best outcome. Remember, once you begin training with the assistive devices, the journey in getting your life back truly begins. Understand there will be pain and it will take perseverance and sheer guts, so do your best to endure—and be strong.

Using assistive devices at first can be daunting and even scary. Crutches are a mainstream assistive device for most leg, foot, and ankle injuries. However, what most caregivers do not take into consideration is crutches aren't always practical, especially for long periods or distances, causing pain and risk of further injury. Walkers are useful, yet over time and through continued use, can become rickety and sometimes unsafe. Remember, walkers and crutches are good alternatives but can be difficult to use on stairs, so ask to be shown proper techniques to maneuver them safely. Always ask for help for proper instruction and practice with any assistive device before using.

The most used and common device for a lower limb amputee is a wheelchair, which is essential for mobility, transport, and travel. You will need a wheelchair soon after surgery, so inquire about getting one as soon as possible. When considering a wheelchair, you must evaluate the accessibility of your home along with the floor plan to determine the need for an installation of a wheelchair ramp and other accommodations with your home. A wheelchair is a necessity that will provide comfort, rest, and mobility as you heal and move toward a new prosthetic.

One vital aspect of living as an amputee is the ever-present need to always think ahead and plan your next move physically and with your life. The reality is amputees are a small minority group compared to the rest of the world, who are left to their own devices on how to function in a physically inaccessible world. Recently, I was asked to do a peer visit with an amputee by the name of Jerry S. He was eighty years old and spry but needed to use a cane. Jerry was old-school, tough by nature, and allowed his stubbornness to prevent him from using a cane. His wife told me he came up with every excuse in the world to not use a cane because he thought using one made him appear weak or helpless. Jerry was falling a lot, and not using his cane increased the chance of permanently hurting himself. I spoke to him and did my best to show these devices are made to help you. Don't let pride impede you from using them. There are vast amounts of information about assistive devices for amputees, so ask your doctor, prosthetist, or physical therapist about them to meet your specific needs. Once you recognize their benefit, get proper training on how to use them, practice using them, and you will be able to get mobile and enjoy your life once again.

LOWER LIMB PROSTHETICS

Prosthetics are a necessity for lower limb amputees, and your recovery process should include full preparation for a prosthesis. According to the Amputee Coalition, below-the-knee amputations are the most common, representing 71 percent of dysvascular amputations, which are caused or gained from poor vascular status of a limb, also known as ischemia. With any lower limb amputation, your prosthesis is an immediate means to walk, move, or stand.

However, for most amputees, the thought of a prosthetic is a fearful reality. Many amputees feel intimidated and worried about what others will see. Richelle E. Goodrich, author of *Making Wishes* (2015), writes, "Relax; the world's not watching that closely. It's too busy contemplating itself in the mirror."[2] Being afraid of others looking at you and your new prosthetic is normal. Today, they design prosthetic devices to be visually appealing and not as frightening or ugly as they used to be. However, receiving your prosthetic can be nerve-racking because when first wearing it, it can feel like the world's eyes are upon you. During this critical time you may feel judged or even gawked at. If this happens, be strong and overlook what others do. I compare the prosthetic-fitting process like my first bike ride. Remember that day? You wanted nothing more than to learn to ride that bike but were afraid to do it on your own. Yet the desire to ride overcame the fear, even though you knew you would have some falls in your future. Still, you forged ahead, and guess what? After a few bumps, scrapes, bruised knees, and some falls, you survived. The same goes for getting your prosthetic. The only difference is your attitude and how you approach the process by either being positive or negative—it is up to you. Preparing yourself mentally and physically for your first prosthetic isn't any different from riding a bike—get on, face the situation, and go.

Meeting with your prosthetist the first time can feel like your first trip to the dentist or a doctor. Not knowing what to expect and not understanding the process can leave you full of fear and apprehension. Your prosthetist is there to see you be successful with your prosthesis, and he or she is the person who will construct your prosthetic, work with you one-on-one, and give you the freedom to stand and walk again. A certified and licensed prosthetist will help you get back to the little things like riding a bicycle, driving a car, going shopping, visiting friends, and enjoying activities once again. Getting your life back through these activities helps in unforeseen and positive ways mentally and physically, by helping you reach a quicker recovery. There is glorified liberty in knowing you can get in your car to go somewhere or take a leisurely walk in the park. This represents freedom and major accomplishment. Remember, working with your prosthetist is the surest way to help you get your life back.

Don't be afraid to ask your prosthetist questions. A good prosthetist will help you every step of the way with skill and compassion. They're someone you can trust. However, my prosthetist alerted me to a startling fact that most prosthetists are "thrown to the wolves" and approached with hard mental questions by worried and scared new amputees. This can be difficult for a prosthetist because, unfortunately, most do not have the training and skills to assess a patient's mental status or condition. While a certified prosthetist is trained in all mechanical and scientific methods of prosthetics, most are not fully trained to handle the psychological issues of many amputees.

Studies from the Amputee Coalition, Össur, and Johns Hopkins University have discovered the need to create new, nationwide programs to help prosthetists address the emotional needs of people with limb loss. These programs provide innovative partnerships necessary to better address the health-care needs of amputees. Kendra Calhoun, former president and CEO of the Amputee Coalition, said in a Yahoo News article, "Amputation Coalition and Össur Partner to Improve the Well-Being of Amputees," "While research has shown that a large number of people with limb loss experience depression or other forms of psychological distress, today's standards of care often leave amputees' mental health needs unaddressed."[3] These new programs will provide necessary training and educational resources to enable prosthetists to take a more active role in enhancing their patients' emotional well-being and resilience.

Many prosthetists now recognize the need to work with patients on a deeper emotional level because most amputee patients are worried, frightened, and confused during this traumatic time in their lives. Amputees, especially new ones, are searching for answers to hard questions and the reality is most prosthetists need to be trained in the deeper psychological aspect of amputations. Most prosthetists are sympathetic and compassionate, and many professional therapists and psychologists have discovered the major benefit for prosthetists to learn how to work with amputees on deeper emotional levels, which helps them better understand and enhance the prosthetic-fitting experience.

However, not every person or personality is the same and not every prosthetist is a good fit. "I didn't get along so well with my prosthetist," Mary J., a right-leg below-the-knee amputee, told me during a peer visit. "She just didn't have the compassion for what I was going through." During this process, compassion is a must because understanding leads to enhanced communication and producing better outcomes. Your prosthetist will be an integral part of your life for a long time, so it is vital that the lines of communication stay open so you have a total understanding of the prosthetic process and are able to ask essential recovery questions. Communication breakdown between you and your prosthetist could lead to confusion, fear, frustration, and even anger. Make sure you choose the right prosthetist that meets your personal and physical needs to ensure a positive and healthy prosthetic outcome.

PROSTHETIC LIMB ACCEPTANCE

With prosthesis acceptance, human nature, as we know, is unpredictable. Acceptance of the prosthetic within your life is based upon whether it provides mobility, functionality, and comfort. Yet many amputees base their acceptance solely on whether it hinders their appearance. If the prosthesis is uncomfortable or if it causes pain, most amputees will not use it, which is a part of human nature (and the brain) working at its finest. Our minds are always looking for the path of least resistance, and each of us are trained from an early age to flee from anything that hurts or causes pain. An amputee must see the true benefit of using the prosthesis for it to be effective. However, some amputees prefer to not use their prosthetic and do better without it. Stephen M., a right-arm amputee, told me, "I work best without my prosthetic. It is just easier to find other ways to do stuff." Stephen is part of a group of amputees who say they are more functional without their prosthesis and feel more comfortable without it.

Alternately, there is another group that relies entirely on their prosthetic. "I can't function without my leg," Jimmy J. said when I visited him while in rehab for his left-leg above-the-knee amputation. "It gets me out of that damn wheelchair to freedom," he told me. Most lower limb amputees need their prosthetic to maintain mobility and freedom. Yet like anything mechanical, prosthetic limbs can have problems. Issues with the prosthetic fitting and adjustments can cause pain, rubbing, chaffing, and even blisters. These problems should be addressed by your prosthetist immediately. Don't let the discomfort, pain, or appearance deter you from wearing your prosthetic because adjustments and repairs can be made to ensure comfort and reliability.

During the first few months of receiving your prosthesis, you will work closely with your prosthetist on the development, sizing, and fitting of the device. A prosthetist's job is to help ease problems and treat any issues that arise before, during, and after with your prosthesis. Daily use of your prosthesis increases the risk of wear and tear and mechanical malfunctions which could deter you from using and wearing your prosthesis. Don't let it. If there is something wrong with your prosthesis, see your prosthetist or doctor right away. Remember, each day you will grow more accustomed to your prosthesis, and soon wearing it will become as routine and easy as putting on a shirt or a pair of shoes.

Prostheses should be designed for comfort and stability, and choosing a prosthetic that fits your lifestyle is an important decision and one not to be taken lightly. This is where being open with your prosthetist about what you want to do and hope to accomplish with your life is essential. Only you know what is best for you, so do not settle on a specific prosthesis unless it provides the necessary functionality to return to a normal life.

Major benefits of the proper prosthesis are being able to get back to your specific lifestyle and life goals. Prosthesis adaptation is critical to help you start enjoying your life by getting back to what you love to do. Talk to your prosthetist about your lifestyle and discuss the things you enjoy doing along with any plans you have for the future. This will help your prosthetist tailor a prosthetic that best fits your lifestyle. If you are an active person, you will need a flexible, more durable prosthetic that will hold up under stress and is designed to undergo the rigors of sports, heavy work, or other physical activities. To accommodate this, some amputees ask for more than one prosthesis: one for sports, such as running, hiking, and skiing, and the other for normal daily use, such as walking or driving. There are some prostheses designed only for water, which can be worn when bathing or swimming. Talk openly about what you intend to do with your life.

Follow the responsible course of action and choose the right prosthetic to fit your lifestyle. The feeling you get from the right prosthetic is immeasurable because once you become acclimated to using it, your world will open to new possibilities never imagined. The extra time and effort in adapting to the prosthesis will pay off for years to come. Using your prosthetic daily gives you the life you once had: enjoying friends and family and getting back to work and the activities you once loved.

Driving: Back Behind the Wheel

It doesn't matter what road you are on, just hold on tight
and enjoy the ride.

—Unknown

*E*very one of us, at some point in our lives, has had a dose of "car
fever." Do you remember wanting desperately to get behind the wheel
and learn to drive? As we mature, our world expands beyond comic
books, bicycles, scooters, and skateboards, and most of us need to
spread our wings and get out on the open road. Having a driver's license
is an avenue to independence, freedom, and doing what you want.

The same applies as an amputee because having freedom after limb
loss can be compared to the same exciting feelings you had as a teenager
finally getting your driver's license—maybe even more so because now
your life has changed, and newfound freedom awaits as you return to
being behind the wheel. Driving once again will be a show of independence and evidence you are taking positive steps and moving forward
with your life. Today, the hustle and bustle of our daily lives makes it
almost necessary to drive a car, such as going shopping or to the doctor, running errands, taking vacations, or just getting out of the house.
As a new amputee, driving could once again be an integral part of your
recovery, independence, and normal lifestyle.

However, whether you are an upper or lower limb amputee,
learning to drive again could be an immense challenge with different
obstacles to overcome. Depending on your limb loss, you may face
learning how to drive in ways you're not used to. It will take practice
operating the vehicle safely by having to learn alternative ways to oper-

ate the vehicle. Relearning old skills could be hard emotionally. During my recovery, I questioned if I would ever get behind the wheel again. *Could I drive with my missing left leg?* I wondered. *Would I have to be a passenger for the rest of my life? Would I have to depend on someone else to get around?* Getting back to driving was important for me for many reasons. Not only did it mean getting my freedom and independence back, but it was another positive step in my overall recovery. Fortunately, since I lost my left leg, I could drive normally and knew when I got behind the wheel during my recovery, I was one of the lucky ones.

Perhaps your amputation prevents you from returning to driving the way you used to. The good news is most amputees return to driving, yet whether you are an upper or lower limb amputee, you may need to relearn new skills and how to operate different equipment. Learning new ways to operate your vehicle may require working with disability driving specialists. These professionals are trained to assist people with disabilities to get back behind the wheel. Research different disability driving specialists in your area. ADED (www.aded.net) is a national organization and database of disability driving specialists around the country.

The big question you may be asking is, can you still drive a car? The answer is yes. According to an article in *ScienceDirect* (2001), over-all, 80.5 percent of participants in their study could return to driving an average of 3.8 months after amputation, although the majority reported a decreased driving frequency. Subjects with left-sided amputation had significantly fewer concerns about driving, while those with a right am-putation frequently required vehicle modifications (40.6%) or have to switch to a left-foot driving style for braking (81.3%) and accelerating (65.6%).[1] Around the globe, hundreds of thousands of amputees have regained their independence by driving once again—and you can, too.

Today, technology has advanced immensely with systems and devices to help amputees drive once again. There are many modified systems designed for amputees to return to driving and normal day-to-day activities. Yet at first, many amputees avoid getting behind the wheel because of fear, not understanding, or lack of confidence. Many worry they will hurt themselves or someone else, and these concerns and feelings are normal. Research has shown that people with all levels of upper or lower extremity amputation can still safely drive a car. Consult with your doctor, physical therapist, or prosthetist about driving when you feel comfortable and able. Make sure you receive the green light from your health-care team before getting behind the wheel. Consult with them on any necessary car modifications adapted to your specific limb loss and prosthetic needs. You may even enlist the help of an occupational therapist or other health-care professional to help retrain for the physical requirements needed to operate a vehicle.

Most amputees adapt well to driving with their prosthesis, and there are others who feel comfortable behind the wheel without the use of their prosthesis. My right-leg amputee friend Tony S. told me during a peer visit, "Man, I was ready to get back on the road. I needed it to feel good again. But I had to make some changes and drive with my left leg. It was tough, but I got the hang of it."

LOWER EXTREMITY AMPUTEE DRIVING

Left Leg: Above- or Below-the-Knee Amputation

If you are a left-leg below- or above-the-knee amputee, driving may not be problematic with any automatic-transmission vehicle. A standard automobile is designed to be operated with the right foot for the gas and brake. However, I have discovered, being a left-leg amputee, there is a slight difficulty getting in and out of the car with your prosthetic or prosthesis. Step in first with your right leg and then pull your residual leg in once seated.

Right Leg: Above- or Below-the-Knee Amputation

Losing a right leg above or below the knee does present a more difficult challenge in driving. In these cases, there will be necessary modifications to reconfigure the gas pedal of your vehicle, such as placing the gas pedal on the left side of the brake pedal and remembering that will be necessary on any new car you purchase for the rest of your life. Ask the salesperson when shopping for a new car about these types of modifications. Remember, if you have trouble adjusting to this change, there are other modifications such as installing hand controls to operate your vehicle.

Amputation of Both Legs and Feet—Full or Partial

Losing both legs is a major traumatic event and returning to driving could be a significant challenge for you. The good news is advancements in modification equipment such as designed hand controls are available to help you get back on the road. Remember, these modifications will be necessary in every vehicle you own and something to always consider when buying a new vehicle. My good friend Morris H., a double amputee who lost both of his legs in a boating accident, has two children he must take care of. His wife died from cancer two years before his boating accident, so he is raising his children on his own. "I had to get back to driving," Morris said. "My kids needed to get to school, and I had to get to work and stuff to do. There wasn't any way we could do life without me driving." So Morris worked hard to learn new driving skills using modified hand controls. There are different hand-control systems are available, such as:

- Hand controls (braking and accelerating)
- Automatic Transmission
- Hand-Operated Dimmer
- Emergency Brake Extension

Hand-control systems contain hand levers to speed up or brake the car with the left hand. The left lever frees up the right hand for signals and operating the gear shifter. Along with the left-hand lever system, other modifications are available, such as a steering knob or wheel spinners that will allow you to steer with either hand. As mentioned before, as a bilateral amputee, speak to a disability driving specialist for the best recommendations necessary for you to return to driving. Research the costs of these modifications, and shop around for the best estimates. There are many companies around the country that specialize in vehicle modifications for disabled, handicapped, and amputee communities. You can research organizations that specialize in vehicle conversion standards, such as the National Mobility Equipment Dealers Association (nmeda.com).

UPPER EXTREMITY DRIVING

Amputation of Hand or Finger or Arms (above and below the Elbow)

If you have lost an arm or hand, modifications are available but possibly not necessary depending on your specific limb loss. With your prosthesis or residual limb, you may operate the vehicle with only small modifications. Consult a disability driving specialist about your specific situation. Could you operate the car using a steering wheel knob or spinner? Is your grip strong enough to maneuver the steering wheel or operate the levers? If the answer is no, specific modifications may be necessary on your vehicle. There are different systems and modifications for hand and finger amputees such as:

- Automatic Transmission
- Changed Gear Shifter
- Changed Secondary Controls (dimmers, wipers, turn signals)
- Changed Steering Device
- Easy-effort steering mechanism
- Chest Strap

Research and discuss with a disabled driving specialist your specific limb loss and about the modifications necessary that will fit you and your lifestyle. Using these types of vehicle alterations provide you with support, confidence, and, most of all, levels of safety driving with one hand. Also, depending on which arm or hand you lost, there may be a need to have proper dashboard controls installed to operate turn signals, horn, headlights, and wiper blades.

Amputation of Both Arms and Hands

This may be hard to believe, but you can get behind the wheel after losing both arms and hands. Significant modifications such as various foot-steering systems can be installed. However, with these systems there is necessary and extensive training required to get behind the wheel. The foot systems allow full control of the car along with steering of the vehicle. Installing these systems is complex and can be expensive, so talk to your occupational therapist and any disability driving specialist about different systems along with financing options available to fit your budget. The systems are high-tech and complex yet deliver a safe and enjoyable driving experience. Modifications of advanced equipment are available for some vehicles, not all. Different systems available are:

- Reduced effort steering system
- Servo Brake and Accelerator system
- Joystick-driving-system modifications
- Swivel seats
- Wheelchair lifts

An article published by the National Highway Traffic Safety Administration (NHTSA) in January 2019 discusses the approximate costs associated with modifying a vehicle:

A new vehicle modified with adaptive equipment can cost from $20,000 to $80,000. Therefore, whether you are changing a vehicle, you own or purchasing a new vehicle with adaptive equipment; it pays to investigate public and private opportunities for financial help. There are however programs that help pay part or all the costs of vehicle modification, depending on the cause and nature of the disability.[2]

One last tip on driving as an amputee: please know that most states require that you register with your local or county DMV about the change in your health and situation. If you do not, you could face fines or even risk being prosecuted if you're involved in an accident caused by your limb loss disability. Please check with your local DMV for advice and guidance on what to do and about any specific requirements in your local jurisdiction. Most amputees qualify for handicapped parking, so inquire about any necessary handicapped placards for your vehicle.

Remember, before driving, check with your local DMV and your state's disability driving laws. Depending on your specific amputation, they may require you to meet with a certified driver rehabilitation specialist before getting back behind the wheel. A driving rehabilitation specialist will assess your driving ability and possibly request a series of evaluation tests that evaluate your reaction time, motor function, and cognitive understanding. These assessments allow your specialist to define any necessary adaptive devices needed for you to drive again. Ask your local DMV about required programs and find a driving rehabilitation specialist in your area. A prescription from your doctor may also be required to obtain any assistive adaptive driving devices for your vehicle. Always check with your DMV on any disabled person permits or about any driver's license changes needed to reflect any restrictions on operating a motor vehicle.

Nevertheless, to drive again, you will have to believe in yourself and be open to learning new ways to drive. It will take a different mindset and willingness to forego how you used to drive in the past, so be patient, retrain your skills, and keep safety at the forefront to operate any motor vehicle. Work hard, be persistent, and, most of all—never give up. Always push forward with all you've got and you'll be back on the road in no time.

Self-Defense and Home Protection

Self-defense is not just a set of techniques; it's a state of
mind, and it begins with the belief that you are worth
defending.

—Rorion Gracie

*O*ne night, as my wife and I were sleeping, there was a loud bang
coming from downstairs. My first instinct was to jump up and see what
was going on. As I sprang forward, I panicked because, for a split second, my brain had forgotten—I had only one leg. As I rushed to put
my leg on, I became nervous as reality hit me. I thought to myself, *How
do you protect your family on one leg? What are you going to do if someone
is downstairs?* I felt extremely vulnerable because I didn't own a gun or
anything notable to protect my wife and myself. Yet I knew I had to
find out what was going on downstairs. Startled, rattled, and confused,
I slowly crept down the stairs. I heard the bang again and my heart
pounded in my chest. As I took another step, I saw something move.
My mind was screaming, *What are you going to do!?* As I came closer to
the moving shadow, the noise crashed around me again. Then I saw it;
was only our porch swing hitting the side of the house because the chain
had broken from a storm's high winds. However, this event opened my
eyes to some hard, cold facts I had to consider. *What if it had been worse,
and an intruder was in the house?*

According to the FBI, violent crimes such as assault, aggravated
assault, rape, kidnapping, home invasions, robberies, and even murder
happen every 24.6 seconds somewhere in the United States. Even

with these kinds of statistics, the odds of you actually experiencing a violent crime is extremely low. However, as an amputee with limitations, protecting yourself should be considered a high priority. Even with violence escalating in today's society, protecting ourselves is often overlooked. Plus, the news media doesn't make many concerted efforts to discuss people with disabilities being at higher risks of violence and even death from intruders or criminals. Criminals perceive people with disabilities as vulnerable and easy targets, more than nondisabled people. As an amputee, and a person with a disability, the question remains: What does crime and domestic violence mean to you?

Whether you are an upper or lower amputee, during your recovery you may find yourself feeling vulnerable and even helpless in certain situations. Anything could happen, and you may be exposed to verbal abuse, psychological abuse, and even physical violence. As a female and even male amputee, being disabled could subject you to unwanted sexual contact, threats, intimidation, and even neglect. During your recovery you could experience your caregivers withholding medications or even destroying or depriving you of your assistive devices. These are terrible aspects to think about, but you must seriously always consider and be aware of these situations to protect yourself and your family. An article published in 2012 by the World Health Organization said that adults with mental impairments are the most vulnerable, with 4.6 times the risk of sexual violence than their nondisabled peers.[1]

Based on the systematic review of violence against adults with disabilities published in February 2012, it was found that disabled people are 1.5 times more likely to be a victim of violence than those without a disability.[2]

Further, according to reports from the Centers for Disease Control (CDC), violence is a severe problem in the United States. From infants to the elderly, it affects people in all stages of life. In 2017, over nineteen thousand people were victims of homicide and over 1.7 million people treated in hospital emergency rooms for an assault-related injury. The number of violent deaths and injuries is just part of the story as increased violence and crimes erode communities by reducing productivity, decreasing property values, and disrupting social services.

Crime and violence can come in many unforeseen forms and lead to confusion, stress, and deep emotional scars. For example, what if during your early days of recovery you discover an individual stealing from you? What if you find things missing? These are hard topics to bring up if you suspect a certain person. Worrying that you're wrong can be intense, so how can you approach that person about your concern? Most criminals, when approached about their wrongdoing, respond in anger, and you could find yourself in a threatening situation. To avoid having this in your life, here are a few things you can do to protect yourself:

- Remove all sizeable sums of money from your home. Secure any valuables and put them in a safe place such as a home safe or a locked cabinet. You could also take a trip to your bank and store your valuables in a safe deposit box.
- Ask this person to leave and never come back to your home. If they do not leave, call the police.
- Protect yourself during your recovery by not being manipulated into giving someone complete access to your home. Guard your personal things.
- Never allow anyone to be in the home when you are not.
- If you feel that this person is stealing from you and you want them to leave yet are afraid of a violent confrontation, have a trusted friend or family member there or call the police to come and handle the situation and remove this person from the premises.

Protecting yourself as an amputee is essential in today's society. There is a lot we can learn to protect ourselves and family from harm. There are many specifically implemented self-defense tactics for people with disabilities that you can put into action against an aggressive attacker. They design these protective tactics for anyone, especially amputees, to make an intruder's strength and size meaningless.

Lions of the African plains spend sixteen hours a day lounging and sleeping in the shade. Yet when night falls, they're hungry and ready to hunt. The ravenous pride hunts everything from gazelles, zebras, hyenas, and buffalos and they work strategically to locate a weak calf or injured animal in the herd. Why? Injured or more debilitated animals are perceived as vulnerable prey because they are slow and cannot protect themselves. The lions attack because they see the animal as a quick meal.

Criminals see people with disabilities the same way—vulnerable, weaker, and not able to defend themselves—making us easy targets. Assailants attack people with disabilities to boost their low self-esteem, and it doesn't matter who you are—today's society forces you to constantly survey your surroundings to keep you safe. You must be on guard everywhere you go, including the grocery store, playground, mall, movie theater, park, bank, and even in restaurants. Be on the lookout for anything that doesn't seem right. Trust your instincts, and if someone or something doesn't feel right, get away from that situation as soon as possible. Awareness and being alert is the most effective weapon you have in protecting yourself.

Violent criminals choose people with disabilities, especially amputees, because they seem to be susceptible targets. So if confronted how do you, as an amputee, defend yourself? The primary way is to let potential criminals and assailants know that you are aware of their presence, arm yourself, and be ready to take action and fight back.

My left-leg below-the-knee amputee friend, Joel S., told me about a scary time he experienced. "One night, I was walking through the living room, when I heard the doorknob to the back door turn. I stopped and froze. I could see the intruder's shadow through the window. Fear rattled me because my gun was upstairs and I didn't know what to do. So I yelled at the top of my lungs for my wife to call the police. I could hear the intruder run away. But the fear gripped me because I felt vulnerable and helpless being on one leg without my gun for protection."

Do what you can to let an assailant know you are not afraid. Stand firm, project strength, and show power either through stance or your voice. Sadly, if you appear weak and helpless, you will most likely become a victim. If you find yourself in a dangerous situation, take a deep breath, use common sense, and always think it through. Do not be stupid, a hero, or get yourself hurt or even killed. Judge the situation, and if the assailant is dead set on robbing you, let them. You can replace material things and valuables, but you cannot replace your life. However, there are certain factors every criminal wants to avoid at all costs. Remember, these eminent facts about most criminals to save your life:

1. Criminals want to avoid getting hurt.
2. Bad guys will do anything not to get caught.
3. Bad guys want things to be quick so they can get away.

As a potential victim, if you show strength and expose any bad person to any of these risks, they will most likely see *you* as a problem or threat and will leave you alone.

The late American journalist Jeff Cooper said in his book, *Principles of Personal Defense,* "The criminal does not expect his prey to fight back." And Jeff also wrote, "May he never choose you, but, if he does, surprise him."[3] So if you are in a position where you feel you are being targeted by a criminal or feel you and your family are in danger, here are some self-defense tactics that will help in protecting you and your family.

Be alert and aware of your surroundings. Have protection near you or on your person, and be prepared to use it. Pick what you are most comfortable with such as a gun, knife, baseball bat, taser, stun gun, mace, or even pepper spray. (Please note that not all these items are legal in every state and many cannot be carried on an airplane.) Research and find out about any permits or licenses necessary to use and carry these on your person and when traveling. Stay vigilant and be aware of anything or anyone out of the ordinary. When confronted, use powerful body language and be direct and assertive by displaying yourself confidently through posture, stance, and strong demeanor. All of this has a dramatic effect by sending a loud signal (I'm not weak. I'm ready to act.) to any adversary. If someone is near and is threatening, project direct and firm verbal boundaries. Shout and raise your voice to be authoritative, which might attract attention from any passersby or potential witnesses in the area. Raising your voice draws attention, which criminals do not want. The closer an assailant gets to you, remember to make your voice louder and do your best to move and get away. Projecting authoritative volumes should warn any bad guy you will not lay down and be an easy target. Shout loudly if they come to close or try to grab you.

Self-defense becomes hands-on when you must fight off an attacker who is trying to rob, choke, stab, or shoot you. If you find yourself in any of these situations, here are a few tips to use:

- Verbal demonstration: use your voice to deescalate a situation and attempt to calm things down.
- Striking the assailant with a hammer fist (if possible): this forward hammer motion can be done sitting or standing.
- Strike the assailant with an object: use any object on your person such as your keys, a small flashlight, a sharp pen or pencil, or a roll of quarters, if necessary. Always carry a tactical object on you.

- Brazilian jiujutsu and some basic striking techniques with hands or feet: you can learn these techniques from most self-defense classes. However, these techniques may not be an option, depending on your arm/hand function.
- If the assailant points a gun, do your best to get away and shout to anyone nearby for help.

Most importantly, be smart and understand your limits by knowing definitively what you're willing to tolerate before you act. Once your tolerance level has been broken, quick and aggressive action is imminent; you must know what you are prepared to do. Are you prepared to inflict pain or physical harm if in a position of being harmed? You must decide and, most of all, never back down. You can't have second thoughts because hesitation could mean life or death. Prepare yourself mentally to protect yourself and your family by any means necessary. Remember, criminals don't want to get hurt and they sure don't want to get caught. Any injury you inflict will, in most cases, cause bleeding, and trauma skyrockets the assailant's chance of getting caught. Remember, lions can't hunt if they are hurt, so they leave their prey alone.

Make awareness your number one security measure. Self-protection starts with having a keen understanding of what is going on around you and within your surroundings: Always examine exits, pathways, hallways, and evacuation plans. Plus, self-protection is also knowing who's around you, what they are doing, and if they make you feel uneasy. The key to awareness is to adopt a preemptive or proactive mindset rather than a reactive approach to personal security. Remember, as you are healing in your recovery you will not have all your strength and are at a slight disadvantage to any criminal who may be stronger or faster. If strength, flexibility, and mobility are concerning issues, be smart and adopt skills of increased avoidance, awareness, and most of all prevention. Your limb loss may not give you the capability to escape from a violent situation or to be physically prepared to confront an intruder or criminal face-to-face. The best defense is to use knowledge as a dangerous weapon by understanding how criminals think, know their deterrents, and arm yourself with proper protection and by completely being always aware of your surroundings.

Do your best to avoid situations where you must use harmful tactics of self-defense. Getting into any physical altercation should be the last resort, so use every means available to thwart it. However, if it comes down to protecting you and your family and you must harm someone, make sure you are prepared to follow through. Always go with your gut feelings and trust your natural instincts. Just like the lions and the animals on the African plain, intuition is the most potent weapon at your disposal. Learn how to apply this human behavior to protect yourself, because intuition does you no good if you are oblivious to what's going on around you. Be prepared, stay alert, remain ready to defend yourself because your life or your family's lives may depend on it.

VI

MAKING THE
IMPOSSIBLE POSSIBLE

• *15* •

Getting Back into Your Life

Hard work spotlights the character of people: some turn up their sleeves, some turn up their noses, and some don't turn up at all.

—Sam Ewing

$\mathcal{I}$s this you? Perhaps you lost your job because of your limb loss that resulted in a significant financial loss? Maybe while you are recovering your medical bills and other financial factors have accumulated and you are overwhelmed beyond measure?

Financial stress is a common problem among many amputees and people with disabilities. A quote I found by U.S. General William Howard Arnold struck a chord with me. General Arnold once said, "The worst bankrupt is the man who has lost his enthusiasm. Let a man lose everything in the world but his enthusiasm and will come through again to success."[1] Money woes can exhaust your energy and your will. Your job is to not let that happen. Remember, money is money, but your health and mental well-being mean more than any medical bill.

Most people who file for bankruptcy have stated that major illness or traumatic accidents that led to disability or amputation are the number one factor contributing to their financial woes. According to a study published in March 2018, the *American Journal of Public Health* found that 530,000 families suffer bankruptcies each year linked to illness or high medical bills.[22] Bankruptcy debtors reported that medical bills contributed to 58.5 percent of bankruptcies while illness-related income loss contributed to 44.3 percent of the many who filed for bankruptcy.

Studies have shown that many middle-class families have faced job loss from an illness that involves high medical insurance copays and demanding deductibles file for bankruptcy.

You will undergo throughout your life medical treatments, including new prosthetics, accessories, checkups, and emergency room visits, and you may encounter financial problems. If you find yourself in need, talk to your health-care team, such as your doctor or social worker, or ask a friend or family member to refer you to someone who could help you with your finances.

Protect yourself by safeguarding your expenses and keep spending to a minimum. Do your best to save money for a rainy day and any unforeseen emergency. When you are in trouble, don't worry about pride. Reach out to someone and ask for help because there isn't any shame in asking for financial help with good intent until you return to work.

RETURNING TO WORK

Getting back to work after limb loss is merely a question of when and if you can return. Everyone's medical condition and recovery time frame are different, and studies have shown that the return-to-work rate for amputees is at about 66 percent. The percent of lower limb amputees who return to the same occupation is 67 percent. Other studies have found that 99 percent of upper limb amputation patients find they must change their career.

These stats are a clear indication that getting back to work involves many variables such as specific limb loss, nature of the work, and physical aspect of the job. Maybe you feel ready to return and get started once again, or perhaps you are experiencing massive amounts of anxiety and stress about returning to work? Do you have doubts about being able to do your job again? Do you fear what others will think of you when you return?

George Addair, a real estate developer during the Civil War, said, "Everything you have ever wanted is on the other side of fear." These words hold true for so many, especially amputees, because fear of getting back to work can cripple and be debilitating. However, returning to work should be your goal, and the way to overcome the fear is through tenacity, ingenuity, self-drive, and a powerful belief in yourself.

We all must work to pay the bills, and getting back to work is a necessity to support our families, especially after limb loss. Mark S., my amputee friend who worked construction, lost his right arm and left leg below the knee in a car accident. He said, "I had to get back to work. I have my babies to feed so I worked my guts out to get back up on two feet to earn a paycheck. Our bills were piling up, and they overwhelmed my wife to tears. But I knew I couldn't do the work I used to do, so I had to get another plan." Mark is a perfect example of using the love for his family as motivation to get going and pursue another career. C. S. Lewis once wrote, "Hardships often prepare ordinary people for an extraordinary destiny."[3] Whatever your motivation, don't back down and never quit. Remember, getting back to work will have an immediate impact on your family, and if you discover your limb loss prevents you from doing the job you used to do, explore other options and find something you can do.

Here is a checklist to help in determining if you can return to your previous work or not:

1. Evaluate if you can physically do the work.
2. Talk to your doctor and prosthetist to help determine if the work you once enjoyed is physically possible.
3. If the possibility is there, check with your human resources department to develop a plan of return.
4. If it's not a possibility, devise a "plan B" on another career path and put it into action.
5. Do you have qualifications for another type of job or position within the company?
6. What qualifications do you have for another career?
7. Are you able to go back to school or learn another trade?

Financial strain can place you under undue stress and make you feel pushed in getting right back to work. However, the strain becomes worse if you find out you can no longer do the work you once did. If you are the breadwinner of your household, without working, finances can get tight, which causes major stress that can lead to depression and feeling hopeless. The intense pressure and angst to return to work can get overwhelming. However, give yourself a mental break, do your best to be patient, take your time, and go back only when you feel it's right.

Depending on your limb loss, you may face the reality of not being able to return to the work you previously did. If so, take the time to soul-search and decide on something else exciting that you want to try. Don't let financial strain and pressure steer you into a wrong decision. These major decisions on a new career are never easy, although extremely important. If this is you, look at it positively as this may be the opportune time to pursue a lifelong dream or another career. Study different options such as going back to school, learning a new trade, and/or furthering your education in another field. Seize the opportunity to improve yourself professionally.

FEAR OF REJECTION ON THE JOB

Being able to return to your job after limb loss is a momentous occasion and one to be celebrated. Most of your coworkers will be curious and excited that you will come back; however, there may be other coworkers who don't understand your limb loss and do not know what to expect. Some people may shy away and not know what to say because of the way you look, or they simply do not know how to accept the change in your body. These are all natural human reactions. So what can you do to help the situation? Do your best to make coworkers feel comfortable by being open and let them know it's okay to talk about your limb loss. Perhaps ask for a company meeting where you can address all your coworkers and their questions to relieve their concerns. If you are a private person, you can express your concerns with your employer and ask your employer for help in talking with your coworkers. Remember, if plausible, it is best to be open and explain about your limb loss, any limitations, and what you are now dealing with. Discuss your additional needs and be open to your coworkers and their feelings about your loss. Provide tips and tricks you've discovered on your limb loss that can help ease uneasiness and tension among your coworkers, which can also help with your own feelings of inadequacy and awkwardness.

When I meet new people, I often address the apparent "elephant in the room" up front, which is my prosthetic leg. For me, it is easier to get it out of the way and help people feel at ease around me. I will make a light-hearted joke, or I'll come right out and say, "I have a prosthetic leg, in case you didn't notice." But I say it in a non-confrontational, even slightly humorous way to ease any apparent tension. In most circumstances, it works like a charm.

Let coworkers know that you will work through your recovery, and as time goes by, you will need less and less of their help. Reaffirm their help and reassure them that the situation is not forever, and you will carry your own workload. When your company hires new employees, do your best to introduce yourself and let them know about your amputation. As life goes by, we often forget that new people may not understand how to interact with you. Talk to them upfront and let them know so they can adapt and sort out their feelings to avoid conflict.

HANDLING INSULTS AND REJECTION AT WORK

Right after my limb loss, going out in public was something I feared. I was afraid of what people thought of me and my prosthetic. One afternoon I stopped for coffee and noticed some teenagers hanging around. As I stood in line, I noticed one of the boys staring at me. Out of nowhere, and to my surprise, he and the others chuckled, all directed toward me. This hurt and I instantly became furious. Yet I knew I had to control the anger, so I ignored them. The world is harsh, yet as amputees, it seems to be harsher than for most because of the insults from people. Insults damage our self-confidence and self-esteem and over time can make you feel alone, alienated, and even angry, which leads to depression and anxiety. Insults and put-downs can become physical, yet most are nonverbal. Facial expressions, such as stony stares, raised brows, and snickers, can all be perceived as direct insults. They can also be jokes or negative comments, mimicry, and fake fascination with your amputation.

Standing up for yourself and not putting up with insults is essential. Sadly, there are those people who will inadvertently make inappropriate comments at work or in public about you. I had a friend named Sean S. who was insulted indirectly. He had lost both of his legs from a terrible tractor accident and had a lawsuit against the tractor company. I overheard some coworkers tell him, "Boy, you are lucky you lost your legs. You are going to make millions." I saw the look on Sean's face. It hurt him. The tractor had rolled over his legs, trapping him for over five hours before help arrived. Sean looked at them, and I'll never forget what he said: "No amount of money can bring back my legs. Don't you ever say that to me again!" Sean had been through a harrowing experience and definitely didn't deserve the insults, even if they came as half-hearted jokes. People can insult you unintentionally through efforts to make you feel better and help you and others do it intentionally, behind your back, or boldly to your face with insults that make for a volatile environment at work. In these situations do your best to be patient and be the judge of your tolerance level. It is your discretion what is acceptable in the work environment. If the insults persist, speak to management and ask for something to be done. No one should have to work in a volatile work environment with people making fun or insulting them.

FEAR OF REJECTION WITH NEW OR POTENTIAL JOBS

Getting back into the workforce means searching for a new job, yet after limb loss it could prove difficult because of fear of rejection or ridicule. Fears of being inadequate or not being able to perform a new job can be stressful, and fear of rejection can overwhelm when interviewing for a new job. Stand firm on who you are when interviewing with a potential employer. If you possess the skills, knowledge, and education to do the job, then go for it. Trust in yourself to do your best to take the focus off your limb loss when in the interview. A good potential employer will see your skills and look past your amputation. Be confident, not arrogant, and believe in yourself to overcome any fears of rejection from potential employers. Remember, you are still the same person before your limb loss, and if you know you can perform a specific job, everything should work in your favor. The key is standing firm and believing in yourself.

If things go awry and you don't understand why, possibly there is more than meets the eye with the potential employer. There are laws that protect amputees and people with disabilities from employer discriminating. The Americans with Disabilities Act of 1990 (ADA) prohibits discrimination and ensures equal opportunity and access for persons with disabilities. "Equal opportunity" is the key phrase to remember because as an amputee you want equal opportunity to show you can perform your duties without special treatment or embarrassment.

Depending on your specific limb loss, you may have to find a job in a brand-new field. Some limb loss situations prevent you from returning to your occupation before the loss, so finding a new job in a new field can be a daunting task. Disclosing your amputation to a potential employer can be scary and make you fear rejection. When not chosen for the job, even though you have the skills and talent to perform the work, it may make you feel discriminated against. However, most of the time this is not the case. Still, these are real factors that you may encounter and must consider. The ADA is enacted to protect people with disabilities from discrimination. When setting up an interview, explain up front that you are an amputee and express your abilities to do specific functions with your limb loss. Never be dishonest about something you think you can do that you can't because in the end it will lead to trouble. In his best-selling book, *Blink*, Malcolm Gladwell said it best: "We don't know where our first impressions come from or precisely what they mean, so we don't always appreciate their fragility."[4]

Being forthright is the best way to approach a potential employer. Be confident in who you are and do your best to make a lasting first impression. A good impression takes the focus from your limb loss and emphasizes the sought-after skills you possess. Thank them for the opportunity and consideration of the new job. These mannerisms go a long way in securing a new job.

With new careers, the most important aspect of being an amputee is recognizing and understanding your potential. Move forward by acknowledging and embracing your new career by remaining focused on the positive things that you can change to make things better. A new career will flourish with acceptance of yourself and adapting to the new life. This is the essential start of a life filled with wonderful and exciting things. Throughout your new career always ask for help, whether it's physical or emotional. Put your pride aside and seek help with any type of issue you are experiencing. New careers include new relationships and friendships, so remember, as an amputee, you're no different from anyone else. Believe you can do most everything everyone else can do—only differently.

As you move through life, you may feel the need to pursue a new dream career. If so, allow yourself to embrace the challenge, the possibilities, and always believe you can do it. Never back down when you meet adversity, and let no one (including yourself) stop your dreams. The more you accomplish empowers confidence in yourself and abilities to get the job done. Always be true to yourself and know that you are still the same person, only stronger than ever before.

· *16* ·

Managing the Stairs and Personal Stuff

My advice to other disabled people would be, concentrate
on things your disability doesn't prevent you doing well,
and don't regret the things it interferes with. Don't be
disabled in spirit as well as physically.

—Stephen Hawking

*A*fter my left-leg amputation, and after being in the hospital over a
month, I came home on New Year's Eve 2017, and all I wanted was to
sleep in my own bed. Desperate, I crawled backward up the stairs and
used every ounce of strength I had in my arms to climb up and get into
bed. I was so weak at the end, my wife had to lift and pull my right leg
under me just so I could lie down. It was a moment I'll never forget.

It doesn't take long to recognize the world is different after limb
loss. Whether you are an upper or lower amputee, your environment,
inside and outside, is now something major you need to consider. Your
world has changed, and now everyday elements could present a challenge and difficulty for you. Everything such as stairs, elevators, escalators, elevator buttons, cutlery, credit card slots, parking meters, driving,
or entrances to buildings could prove tough. The outside environment
for any amputee presents challenging obstacles even more than your
familiar household surroundings. As you venture back into society,
everyday common errands and tasks could take on an element of difficulty, such as inaccessible businesses, stores, banks, doctor's offices, and
any other place in your community.

Today's society hums along seemingly at warp speed, and sadly the world does not slow down for people with disabilities. Although programs and laws have been enacted to help remedy these factors, society, in general, is still not convenient nor disability friendly. The Americans with Disabilities Act (ADA) was signed into law by George H. W. Bush in July 1990. The act is a civil rights law that prohibits discrimination against individuals with disabilities in all areas of public life, including jobs, schools, transportation, and all public and private places that are open to the general public. The purpose of the law is to ensure that people with disabilities have the same rights and opportunities as those provided to individuals based on race, color, sex, national origin, age, and religion. Disability accommodation is an essential and viable aspect of ethical business operations. The ADA is there to protect people with disabilities, yet it still doesn't address entirely the immediate challenges in your daily limb loss life. Many businesses are still not accommodating nor accessible for people with wheelchairs, walkers, or prosthetic limbs.

The more you become accustomed to your outside surroundings, the better you'll be at navigating with greater success and independence. Getting around in society is based upon basic techniques required to manage everyday obstacles. Limb loss experts call this "advanced gait training," which are methods of mobility for lower and upper limb amputees. Going up and down stairs is often a necessity and can be done safely with implementing proper techniques. Being in new environments, especially when traveling, pushes you to learn new skills in moving around within your newfound personal environment.

You will discover the outside world is filled with challenges most take for granted such as stairs, escalators, buttons, handrails elevators, ramps, inclines, and different surfaces. Being out in public as a lower limb amputee, or even at home, it's almost unavoidable that you will encounter flights of stairs, hills, and uneven surfaces. To safely maneuver them, you can use an approach that involves a form of *"jackknifing."* This is where you take each step sideways while holding onto the rail with both hands for support. Then there is the *step-by-step method*, which is designed for lower limb amputees who need to climb stairs with or without a railing. This method is the safest way to go up and down stairs. Most people normally step-over-step on stairs; however, lower limb amputees have trouble doing step-over-step because it's difficult to push up, maneuver, and bend with a prosthetic.

The step-by-step method can be used by every lower extremity amputee and can be used on every set of stairs. Start by shifting your body weight from the prosthetic when going up the stairs and use your healthy remaining limb to start up the stairs. Bend your body (trunk) over the sound leg for balance and then follow by bringing the prosthetic leg up on the same step. Hold the rails for safety and repeat the same process on each consecutive level. When using stairs remember, "Up with the good (healthy limb), down with the bad (prosthetic limb)." I'm not saying there is anything wrong with your amputated limb; I only use this as a simple way to remember the steps and motions to maneuver steps safely. When going down the steps, we can apply the same, "Down with the bad." When stepping down, place your prosthetic leg firmly down first. Shift your weight for balance over to your prosthetic and then transfer your weight to your sound leg and step down. Follow though by bringing both legs safely onto the stair tread. Repeat these actions until safely down. Do not attempt to do this fast or you can risk falling. With practice, speed and agility will improve. Monica T., a left-leg below-the-knee amputee, told me during a certified peer visit that the stairs made her nervous. "Yeah, stairs frightened me," she said. "I didn't really know how to manage them. I took my time and was slow at first, but after a while I got my bearings."

Walking in public and maneuvering curbs and crossing the street is a necessity. Apply the same step-by-step technique described for stairs. Remember, "Down with the bad and up with the good." Since curbs are mostly one step instead of many, this should not present a problem for you.

UNEVEN SURFACES:
GRAVEL, SAND, SNOW, AND GRASS

If you are a lower limb amputee, your prosthetist will work with you on specific gait training on uneven surfaces. There are multiple types of surfaces in our world such as grass, gravel, concrete, and snow, along with different terrains such as sand, rock, ice, and even uneven carpet heights. These surfaces could cause significant problems maneuvering over with your prosthesis. The only way to move safely on different surfaces is to do it slow and walk, but always be aware and alert of your surroundings and any uneven terrain. This is critical to avoid slips and falls or risking further injury. If there is a surface you feel unsteady with or fear falling on, avoid it if possible. When in doubt, be safe and make good choices, and avoid conditions and surfaces that you know are problematic for you.

RAMPS, HILLS, AND INCLINES

Going uphill for a lower limb amputee is difficult and can be problematic. However, varying factors come into play when going uphill, such as health condition, age, and specific amputation. They design most prosthetics to not include the mechanical function called "dorsiflexion," which is a "backward bending" movement of the hand or foot which happens in the prosthetics mechanical foot and ankle portion. This is the reason going uphill (ascending) or inclines, ramps, or steep grades are challenging because of this lack of functionality. Going down requires "plantaflexion" in the foot/ankle, which is the movement of your foot "away" or "forward" from your body by bending at the ankle much like a ballerina stands on her tiptoes or when you step and press on the gas pedal. Most prosthesis mechanics are not designed to have this functionality. However, advancements with prosthetic technology has many new prosthetics that address this concern. Using a prosthetic on a hill takes coordination and strength to push yourself up any steep incline. Going down is hard because of the added problem of the person's weight pushing (posterior) on the knee joint and balance, resulting in an abnormal flexion of the knee which could cause a fall or further injury.

To safely maneuver up a steep incline, place your body weight more forward than normal over the prosthetic. This allows the prosthesis to function properly by performing maximal dorsiflexion by keeping the knee or knees in an upright extension suitable to push your body up. When going down, gravity will work against you so you must shift your weight to not pick up speed, causing you to fall. Remember, the faster you go, there is less functionality with plantarflexion. The speed simply gives you less time to properly posture and stance. Be prepared when going downhill to exert a greater-than-normal pressure on the rear wall or "heel" of the prosthesis to have proper knee extension. With plenty of practice, most amputees discover it is easier to go up and down inclines by taking their time and maintaining a strong balance, good posture, and short and equal strides. Visually, most amputees prefer to take shorter strides just as an average person would because the movement looks normal compared to walking fast and displaying an uneven gait.

There are other methods of managing inclines such as *sidestepping*, which allows you to go sideways or zigzag one step at a time. Zig zagging allows you to balance while going horizontally across the incline, moving up one grade at a time. Although this can take longer, some amputees prefer this method as a safer way to tackle an incline.

ENVIRONMENTAL BARRIERS

There are many unforeseen barriers in your environment that once went unnoticed but now are a major concern. Everything from shortage of handicapped spaces to the ever-present problem of handicapped parking spaces located farthest from the entrance of a business. Another annoyance is handicapped parking spaces at state fairs, stadiums, convention, community centers, and even airports miles away from any designated entrance. Then you have "handicapped accessible" hotel rooms assigned (for unknown reasons) furthest away, at the end of long hallways seemingly miles from the nearest elevator. Then there are hotels and motels that do not have inside elevators or room access. This forces lower limb amputees to maneuver large flights of stairs. Still, there are many buildings and businesses that have steep grades, ramps, uneven sidewalks, or steep flights of stairs, making it challenging to enter.

Many places of business lack ample space in front of entryways and doorways for wheelchairs or walkers. And many businesses include entryways with have massively heavy doors, making it hard on upper and lower limb amputees. Swinging doors or rotating doors are still prominent in older, more significant buildings and can be problematic for you as a lower limb amputee. Plus, older buildings (e.g., courthouses, government buildings, post offices) were built to different standards and codes which allowed narrow hallways, making it impossible to pass through for a wheelchair-bound disabled person. As you travel, you will find bathrooms in many rest areas designated as "handicap bathrooms" too small for wheelchairs, making it virtually impossible to access for the disabled. Shopping for clothes can be almost impossible in some retail stores, with all the racks and rows of clothes crammed together in small spaces. All you must do is enter any local big box store and there you will see clothing racks shoved up as close as to one another, leaving no room for a disabled person's wheelchair. These close quarters can also be troublesome for an amputee with a prosthetic. Trying to weave in and out with a prosthetic through the maze of merchandise makes it almost impossible to walk.

Be aware that when you walk into a public office, mall, business, or convenience store, you may find freshly mopped floors which poses a major slip and fall hazard. Evaluate your immediate surroundings and always keep your safety in mind. And many (not all) public transportation vehicles such as buses or trains, and even subway systems, are not adapted for those of us with assistive devices. Just getting into the subway in New York City as an upper or lower limb amputee could be almost impossible with key cards, necessary coins and change, holding objects, and maneuvering flights of stairs, narrow halls, and metal gates.

Almost every mall in American and around the world has escalators. Seemingly innocent and easy to do, escalators for an amputee, upper or lower, can be dangerous, challenging, and downright unsafe. Trying to get on an escalator takes balance and coordination, and with a prosthetic, it can be a major challenge to maintain your balance. If you are an upper limb amputee, getting on and off and getting a secure hold on the moving rail could be problematic, leaving you unsafe and prone to a harmful fall. When boarding an escalator, take your time getting on and off and make sure to always hold the rails, to the best of your ability, to maintain your balance. Remember, it may look like a piece of cake getting on and off an escalator; however, they are extremely dangerous and could cause you to be hurt, so proceed with care and caution.

AMPUTEES USE MORE ENERGY

Even after being fully recovered, don't be surprised if you still feel a reduction in your physical abilities. Maneuvering around within your environment can be hard even after being an amputee for a long time. Why? It is simple physics at work here. People get older and it is harder for most with differing ailments and body conditions. However, lower limb amputees use excessive amounts of energy with their prosthetic to walk compared to a normal person. As an upper amputee, you could see your energy drop drastically when pushing a shopping cart, lifting your purse, carrying baggage, vacuuming, or even doing simple tasks like lifting grocery bags. These are aspects many people take for granted, but for you, an amputee, they can drain your energy fast.

Monica S., a right-arm below-the-elbow amputee, told me, "I get tired even washing dishes." She said, "Using my arm and my stump exhaust me." Studies have shown that upper and lower amputees that use a prosthetic use more energy than others do. A person in a wheelchair will use up to 9% more energy than a person walking on two legs. Below the knee, amputees can use up to 25% more energy compared to a person on two good legs. An amputee missing both legs below the knee, using their prosthesis, can burn up to 41% more energy. And above-the-knee, amputees (unilateral) can spend over 50% more energy than a normal individual. And if you are missing both legs above the knee (bilateral), you can expect to burn over 110% more energy than a normal healthy individual.

TRAVEL, GETTING AROUND, AND PREPARATION

Simple things in your life such as going on vacation or going to necessary appointments in your own community can be extremely difficult. Traveling long distances as an amputee, you must think of ways to save energy to make life easier and allow you to enjoy a stress-free and more comfortable experience. When getting ready to travel within the United States or abroad, consult with your doctor, your prosthetist, or any disability-certified travel agencies in your area to help your trip. There are many companies now dedicated to helping amputees and disabled people with their travel needs. Research different travel agencies and travel touring services and find out precisely what they do to help amputees. The goal with these companies is to design packages tailored to ease stress and include everything for one price. These all-inclusive packages and rates take the guesswork out of how you will get around, have access to places you want to see, and most of all remove the stress by knowing the entire cost of your trip.

Traveling as an amputee can be a challenge, but it is worth the effort to experience new places and enjoy times with friends and family

Today, vacations and resort destinations have stepped up the game to accommodate amputees and people with disabilities. There are now many tours and sightseeing trips available that are more handicap assessable. And even most cruise ships, resorts, or remote destination vacations have taken people with disabilities seriously and ensure all disabled passengers and patrons have equal access to everything on board the vessel and other designated areas. However, remember to speak to the cruise line or travel agent about access to the ship, access inside the ship, and accommodations that fit your limb loss once you are onboard. Ask about cabin sizes, elevator access, hallways, and entryways. Cruise lines build ships to accommodate as many passengers as possible so keep in mind the rooms, hallways and entryways in the lower fare cabins are narrower on the ship.

When planning a trip, remember to dress for adventure and pack smart. Bring comfortable clothing and shoes that fit the locale and allow easy access to put on your prosthetic if needed. Remember, always take care of yourself by periodically checking yourself for any skin breakdowns, and if you're out don't ignore the warning signs of any pain. If you are away from home and start feeling pain, stop and find out what's wrong. If you must, every so often, excuse yourself and check your residual limb for any skin, blisters, or irritation issues.

When you are planning any activity, keep all essential first aid items with you. We all know things happen, so plan for any unforeseen emergencies with you and your prosthetic. When flying, leave nothing in your checked baggage that you can't live without. Keep everything you need (within reason) on your person or carry-on bags. Everything from prosthetic device accessories, device chargers, and any essential medications keep with you because if your checked baggage is misplaced or sent to the wrong destination (it happens often), it may be days before you get it back—if ever. So, keep everything important on your person.

Going through a large airport, train, or bus terminal, even for an average person, can be hard, but for an amputee it can be extremely difficult so allow yourself extra time for any needed disability assistance or checking-in and boarding with your bags. Keep in mind that going through security in airports could take longer because of the sensitive alarms and systems in place. Most security alarms are triggered by many prosthetic devices with different metals and could cause a delay. To prevent this from happening, explain before approaching your situation. This will hopefully save time in getting through.

When your trip has you staying in hotels, remember to request pertinent information about hotel room accessibility in advance. Why? Most (not all) handicapped rooms that are advertised as "handicapped rooms" do not meet handicapped accessible standards and regulations. Unfortunately, even though these facilities promote these rooms to be handicapped accessible, most are not and cannot accommodate wheelchairs or the disabled amputee. Ask about handicapped rooms that are closest to the elevators and conference rooms when you're traveling. Remember, once you are in the room and it doesn't suit your needs, ask for another room or other arrangements to be made if the room doesn't meet your needs. If it is necessary, ask for items of furniture to be moved or removed to make the accommodations work for you.

Many travel destinations, national parks, and resorts are now handicapped accessible. However, it is necessary to find out about any resort or national park area's handicapped accessibility. Research online or ask the local chamber of commerce about local travel guides or organizations for more information.

Moving on with your life involves getting out, being active, travel, and adventure. When visiting an unfamiliar destination, double-check beforehand on available handicapped accessibility of the place you intend to visit. Remember to never allow outside obstacles to prevent you from traveling or moving around in your area. Get out and adapt, improvise, plan, and strategize and enjoy what life offers. Knowing yourself and what you want to do is the vital element in living an active and prosperous life. Every problem you solve on your own, every challenge you face, brings more confidence and inner strength to help you live your best life.

Limb loss life includes always being prepared for every situation and circumstance. Everything such as doing your daily routine, driving to work, taking the bus, riding a train, or even walking in your neighborhood, you need to have extra accessories on hand to ensure your safety and to remain mobile. Depending on your specific health condition and limb loss, carrying essential equipment nearby such as tools or various wrenches for your prosthetic is a must. I use my old prosthetic legs as backups or spares in the car and on trips to ensure I have them in case of a malfunction. All of this applies to upper extremity amputees, and it is smart to have spares on your prosthetics and accessories. I call these *Amputee Emergency Packs*, and these packs have got me out of jams on multiple occasions. Amputee Emergency Packs should include items such as:

- Extra stump socks
- Prosthetic liners
- Regular socks, dressings
- Second-skin bandages
- Gauze
- Antibiotic ointment
- Allen wrenches
- Hex key wrenches (check size on prosthetic)
- Lock-Tite,
- Small bottle WD-40 (for squeaks)
- Shoehorns
- Plumber's tape

Still, use whatever you feel necessary to maintain your mobility and functionality when away from home. Evaluate your basic essentials and gather everything you need daily. Keep it in a backpack, on your person, or in a place you can easily access. You must be prepared for the worst-case scenario; however, you can't be expected to live in fear, but there is a responsibility now in protecting yourself from mishaps. Accessories help with proper routine limb care that is essential daily because of the natural factors associated with prosthetic wearing such as moisture and sweat being trapped in your prosthetic socket and liner. Proper skin care under these conditions is crucial for a long-term outcome of preventing other significant complications. Each day you will develop a routine, and part of that routine should include looking for skin issues such as pressure patches and points. Part of being an amputee involves checking your body for anything unusual, such as distinctive redness or irritated areas. If you discover pressure points, blisters, or irritated areas, they cannot be ignored and seek medical attention as soon as possible. If ignored, these issues could become worse, causing skin infections. A prosthetic liner fits tight and prevents air from getting to your skin and limb. Increased temperature and movement create a moisture-filled environment perfect for harmful bacteria to grow. This bacterium could cause skin infections, breakdowns, rashes, and harmful irritation.

Examine yourself for skin breakdown because skin damage can happen quickly and could lead to other severe complications. Skin damage can start with blisters and could develop into wounds, placing you at risk of more significant health issues. If you are a diabetic and have diabetic neuropathy, always be aware of what is happening to your body. Neuropathy numbs extremities to where you cannot feel the pain of wounds or blisters. This could lead to trouble, so inspecting the skin on and around your body is now essential in your life.

Hygiene and bathing as any amputee can be a challenge. For lower limb amputees it is best to shower or bathe at night before you go to bed because being exposed to hot water your limb will swell, making it harder to put your prosthetic on. If you are an upper limb amputee, you must learn alternative ways to wash and use bottles such as shampoo and shaving cream in the shower. There are products that are designed for upper limb amputees to make showering and bathing easier. When bathing or showering, wash your limb with mild soap and never rub your skin dry with a towel. Always pat dry your skin instead of rubbing to prevent damage to any potential skin-breakdown areas. Before putting on your prosthetic, ensure your residual limb is completely dry to prevent bacteria from growing and causing wound infections.

Be careful using different powders as they can be problematic and should be avoided. Powders such as talcum powder, baby powder, or cornstarch, which is found in products for an athlete's foot, can lead to major problems causing massive irritation. In the moist and sweat-filled environment in your socket, these powders get sticky and dry up, and when the powders dry up, they ball up, causing extensive abrasion, soreness, and redness. There are many lotions approved for healing and use with amputees. For skin care I recommend the following:

- Silicone-based lotions
- Tegaderm
- Neutrogena Body Oil
- Cold-pressed organic coconut oil
- Jojoba oil

As a major part of your daily routine, taking care of your body and skin is an essential task you must never forget to do. Skin breakdown can happen quickly in certain areas so discovering redness, soreness, and skin issues, in most instances, means your prosthetic device needs an adjustment. Avoid eating salty foods and meats which can help with inflammation and skin issues. Too much salt intake can make your limb swell, making it hard for a correct fitting and increasing risk for pressure sores which can lead to infection. If you find your skin breaking down or trouble areas, see your doctor or prosthetist immediately.

Another essential aspect of living as an amputee is daily prosthetic accessory care. Prosthetic device care involves daily usage of various accessories, such as liners and socks—tools vital to your mobility and function. Since you are a new amputee, you must adapt to part of your daily living is maintaining and washing anything that meets your skin. Everything from prosthetic liners, socks, and even the inside of the socket itself can hide germs and bacteria. Use a mild soap and water and make sure everything is dry before use. Prosthetic liners have a lifespan of about 6–12 months, and you can detect when the liner is breaking down by small tears, thin or worn areas, or small and large holes. If you see these things happening, talk to your prosthetist for recommendations on new liners and adjustments. Maintaining your body, your residual limb, and the prosthetic device is essential in living a healthy amputee lifestyle. It all starts with implementing daily routines and applying simple tools will ensure your long-term health.

THE DISCOUNT FOOD DIET

Many amputees find it to be a necessity to penny-pinch and watch their spending to make ends meet. Most people can save money by avoiding buying cheap, unhealthy food such as fast food and junk food. Some amputees require special diets because of health conditions such as weight issues, arthritis, diabetes, osteoporosis, and many other many health problems. These types of health conditions often require more expensive, not-so-budget-friendly food choices to maintain optimal health. Many amputees endure additional expenses such as for prescriptions, assistive devices, treatments, office visits, prosthesis alterations, and modifications to their homes for a suitable living.

If your budget is tight, it may be time to seek alternatives in good food choices from reputable discount stores around the country. A study was performed at the University of Nevada, Las Vegas, and a referenced article written by Haven Nieman, and Keonna Summers found that the quality of fruits and vegetables at dollar stores is just as good as regular grocery store produce.[1] Discount stores exist in most cities across the country and many are an excellent alternative for amputees and people with disabilities to get excellent quality, healthy food. If you are limited with your finances or are in a position where you are struggling, there's nothing wrong with finding discounted produce or goods that provide the same nutritional value.

Shopping for your food may be a challenge because of limited supplies and financing, yet, with perseverance, you should be able to find stores in your area that have the foods you need—but cheaper. And now with the resurgence of grocery stores offering delivery and in-store shopping for customers, plus hands-free pickup, it makes it easier as an amputee to get the foods you need. However, it is good to get out and do your own shopping because there is satisfaction and independence in doing so. But if your condition does not allow you to shop efficiently for yourself, then the online ordering and grocery pick-up or delivery is always the next-best option. And don't discount using a monthly food service such as HelloFresh, Green Chef, or Home Chef where food is delivered to your home, packaged and ready to heat and eat.

Living life as an amputee involves complicated and uncomplicated factors you will have to embrace. As you enter more into your new life, you will discover what works best for you within any situation. With work, play, and traveling, learn all you can about living as an amputee. Use your skills, common sense, compassion, and creativity to forge new paths toward making your life and your dreams a reality. Always remain confident in your endeavors, trust in yourself, and communicate to others your feelings about your life as an amputee. Once you feel the freedom in taking care of yourself, opening up to new challenges, and accepting who you are as the courageous person you've become—your life will flourish beyond your expectations.

· *17* ·

Managing Stares from Others

It was lovely. Not to be stared at, not seen, but being pulled into view by the interested, uncritical eyes of the other.

—Toni Morrison

*P*eople will react in different ways to your limb loss. Some will have compassion, sympathy, or curiosity, and others might be rude, ignorant, or even standoffish. Their reaction is beyond your control, yet how you react is completely up to you. Once you move on with your life, you will experience some eye-opening experiences because your overall prosthetic life involves many critical factors, yet one of the most significant aspects is dealing with people. Life is full of diverse people which makes dealing with different personalities something that is unavoidable, all of which make some interactions extremely difficult. People are inquisitive; however, some do not handle the curiosity of your prosthetic well and will make mistakes when interacting with you. Many people do not adapt easily to change, especially children.

Throughout my recovery, I discovered that my perception of people drastically diminished and changed. I became extremely disappointed with many people in my circle. The disappointment wasn't from what they said or had done; it was from what they didn't say or do. Many ignored me, even forgot me, and the hurt of this reality hit me hard. I asked "WHY" so many times, but the answers seem to never come. I was living a harsh reality, and, over time, these feelings and hurt grew deeper and deeper that I dreaded going out in public. I believed people didn't want to be around me because of the way I looked. Now,

I know this isn't true, and it was all in my mind, but the hurtful reality remained; I was left out and ignored by friends who I never expected would turn their back on me. Since then, I have made many new friends that have helped me recover. My guess is God made room for the right people in my life and took out the wrong ones in one fell swoop.

Over time, don't be surprised to see some people disappear from your life. Sadly, it could be the ones you would least expect. Remember, losing friends is not a reflection on you or how you look. Their absence in your life is their responsibility—and not yours. Not having them in your life is their loss so don't be afraid to let go of these people, but be prepared to have a different view and perception of some.

Going out in public as an amputee may be difficult because of the fear of how people will look at you. There will be some people who may surprise you with their compassion, friendliness, and kindness, and it will not take long for you to judge moral character among those around you. Unfortunately, you will also meet people who are hurtful, say inappropriate things, ask impolite questions, and even make snide or off-color comments. At first, when going out in public with your prosthesis, it may seem as if everyone is staring at you. (Hint: they're not!) And it may appear that the stares are coming from everyone: men, women, and children. It is in these moments where you feel vulnerable, ugly, making it hard and an intense emotional challenge. Sometimes people will come right out and ask what happened to your arm or leg. Then there are those that look the other way as if disgusted and want nothing to do with you. I've seen some people do a double take, then stare at me and my leg unapologetically.

Since I have become an amputee, it seems when I run into certain people, they seem to know all about being an amputee, even though they aren't one. It has amazed me how many people want to let me know their direct experience with amputee family members or friends. I've heard it all, and you will too. Don't be surprised or impatient when people tell you their friend, father, mother, sister, brother, or grandparent had a limb amputated. I believe they earnestly want to tell you their story because, in some weird way, it makes them appear familiar with the subject and to feel more comfortable with you.

To make matters more intense is most of these people read or hear stories about amputees climbing Mount Kilimanjaro, hitchhiking across the country, or running in the Olympics. Don't misunderstand me; these are incredible feats achieved by incredibly talented, spirited, and hardworking amputees who deserve full credit for their accomplishments. My point is that based on these accomplishments, some people think EVERY amputee should be doing these extreme and powerful things, and those who aren't are unmotivated or even possibly a "slacker." Have you climbed Mt. Kilimanjaro? They ask you. "Are you running a marathon, soon?" These questions make it hard, and even though you know these people mean well, these scenarios make it difficult for any amputee. Yet I believe each amputee should use these feats as motivation to pursue their own dreams and achievements, and there isn't anything wrong with that. Again, every time one of these stories hits the airwaves, I have had complete strangers ask me if I've ever done such a feat and even been asked, "Why does your leg not look like the person running in the Olympics?"

When first asked these kinds questions from strangers, you may be taken aback or even resent them. There isn't anything wrong with feeling this way, and it is human nature, but do your best to be understanding and patient. I have a good friend, Jamie D., an above-the-knee amputee who has been dealt a tough hand most of his life. He was orphaned at nine and lived in foster care until he was fifteen. He was adopted into a wonderful family, yet they didn't have the money or means to send him to college. So in adulthood Jamie worked hard in order to give his family the best life he could offer them. He lost his right leg below the knee at work when a steel beam fell from a crane, pinning his right leg. Jamie stepped up and faced the challenges of getting back up on his feet for his family's sake. He worked hard, stayed motivated, and eventually got back to work. To me, stepping back onto a construction site after a terrible accident is the epitome of bravery and tenacity. Sadly, the bravery, an astonishing show of determination, and perseverance such as this doesn't merit the same enthusiasm from the news and media as the other stories mentioned above.

The key is to remember not to fall into the trap of comparison. You are you and cannot be someone else. The goal is to find yourself and discover what you can do best and what you want out of life. Many amputees fall prey to these unrealistic comparisons and attempt to do feats they cannot accomplish. This puts them in harm's way and risk hurting themselves and damaging their health. However, as Thomas Edison once said, "If we did the things we are capable of, we would astound ourselves." American football coach Lou Holtz said it best: "Ability is what you're capable of doing. Motivation determines what you do. Attitude determines how well you do it."

As you get back into the world, do your best not to listen to the "naysayers" and overcompensate by attempting to do things that aren't achievable for you. Keep in mind, these achievements may be accomplished later with hard work, motivation, and fortitude to push yourself to conquer long-term and short-term goals. Yet only you can decide what goals are attainable and reasonable. Remember, if you feel you are ready to meet specific challenges, then go for it. Only do it for you and not for anyone else. Keep the goals and motivation realistic by understanding even though you are still capable, it just may take you longer and an immense amount of work to get there.

People will come forward and offer their help as you get back into normal life. There may be some who, for whatever reason, weren't around when you were going through your early recovery and now that you are getting better want to reengage with you. Even though these people want to help, perhaps you are at the stage where you want to accomplish your goals on your own. This is natural, so when approached, be polite and let them know you are going to do things yourself. If you want help, then accept it. The choice is up to you. Most people have good intentions; however, most personal growth happens by pushing yourself. It's easy to deter someone from wanting to help, yet do your best to not let this happen and be positive by showing your appreciation. There may come a day you need their help.

Confidence goes a long way, especially when handling questions about your limb loss and prosthesis. When people seem inquisitive, stand firm and be confident with your answers. Most people are sympathetic and are curious about something that appears out of the ordinary. Amputation almost always raises curiosity and people will ultimately ask questions. People will be people, yet not everyone reacts the same. Some may stare inadvertently, or others are too timid to ask a question. Others may treat you negatively or even turn their head away and ignore you. In these situations do your best to be patient, keep calm, and answer questions to the best of your ability. Don't let the stares and negativity get to you. Step away and ignore those who act ignorant or nasty.

By being prepared for questions, you will be more comfortable when asked and will know what to say. Most people are curious about how you lost your limb. Many people I've spoken with ask me about my limb loss because someone in their family or one of their friends has undergone an amputation and they are genuinely interested. This is one of the major reasons for this book and why that I became a Certified Peer Visitor (CPV) through the Amputee Coalition. My goal is to help anyone with questions and concerns about being an amputee.

At a recent visit to my prosthetist for a routine checkup, I met Stephen W., a right-leg below-the-knee amputee who had just lost his leg and was still in his wheelchair. Stephen looked at me and my prosthetic and opened up without hesitation. "I'm here getting my first prosthetic leg," Stephen said. I immediately realized an especially important fact. There is a sovereign camaraderie among amputees, and I believe it comes from the fact that each of us understands the pain and perseverance each of us has undergone—and survived. It appears to almost be a rite of passage, a gateway into knowing the person inside, because amputation, losing a part of one's body, is the truest test of inner integrity, strength, and willpower. Stephen opened up more and asked, "How long did it take to get used to your prosthetic?" I was happy to answer his question, and we then talked about his situation. I helped him and his wife understand the next steps and what to expect. I am always open to questions from other amputees because it has been a true honor in getting to know some wonderful people around the country and learn more about amputation.

QUESTIONS FROM CHILDREN

One hot summer day my family wanted to go swimming. It petrified me at the thought of what people were going to think of me and my missing leg, yet I mustered up the guts to get in the water. I took off my prosthesis, exposing my stump, and thought self-consciously that everyone was staring at me, but I got in the water. Later, as I was getting out of the pool, a little boy came over, stopped, and stared at me. He innocently asked, "What happened to your leg?" His mother shouted at him not to bother me, but I told her it was alright. "My leg was really sick, and it had to be removed," I replied calmly. The little boy swam away, satisfied with my answer. In that fleeting moment, I discovered that most children have an innocent curiosity about limb loss.

Children, by human nature, are curious about things they do not understand, but unlike adults, they are uninhibited and see no problem in asking questions. However, don't be surprised about awkward stares or odd questions from young people. Most do not mean any harm by any of it or by staring at you. They're only inquisitive about your missing limb because they are just not used to seeing people in this way. When a child stares at you (it will happen), remain composed before speaking and keep in mind they're only reacting naturally from the way they have been taught. However, you do not have to allow a young person to belittle you or treat you disrespectfully.

During a certified peer visit, I met with Thomas J., a right-leg above-the-knee amputee, an army veteran of Iraq. He told me about the time, right after he had come home from the war, that he had a run-in with a group of rude teenagers in a mall. "I walked by and I heard two boys snicker," he said. "Normally, I would have ignored it and walked on by, but on that day, I wasn't having it. So I stopped dead in my tracks and asked, 'You boys have a problem?' The boys looked surprised and unsure of what to do or say because they didn't expect me to react. I stood still with a dead stare as the boys quickly walked away."

No one must endure such behavior from anyone. If this happens, do your best not to react emotionally and end up making a mistake, getting into trouble, or hurting someone. Leave, collect your thoughts, and use common sense in these situations.

Do your best to be approachable when you encounter people. Be open and willing to talk about your loss, which helps in gaining in-depth insight and supportive perspectives from others. Talking and answering questions allows you to help others and yourself in self-discovery. Take it upon yourself to be there for others because there are many people who suffer from deep emotional and physical pain from their disabilities. Many people hide their guilt and shame because for fear of exposing their inner feelings and showing weakness by asking for help. I see amputees and disabled people as powerful warriors existing in an able-bodied world. Awareness and acceptance of who you are as a person, enduring an eye-opening, gut-wrenching reality—living with limb loss—is a personal and gratifying acknowledgment of who you truly are and the heart, soul, and essence of living life as an amputee.

• 18 •

The New You

Making the Impossible Possible

> If you can't fly then run, if you can't run then walk, if you
> can't walk then crawl, but whatever you do you have to
> keep moving forward.
>
> —Dr. Martin Luther King

*P*erhaps throughout your life you have been pursuing your dreams, and losing a limb may seem like an insurmountable obstacle keeping you from achieving them. Limb loss doesn't have to stop you. Embrace the challenge by recognizing that you can accomplish anything you set your mind to. The difference is something small, seemingly insignificant, yet large in its effect, and that is—your attitude. Staff Sergeant Travis Mills is a quadruple amputee whose body was shattered when a bomb took away all four limbs. He bravely told his harrowing life story in his video, *Travis. A Soldier's Story.*[1]

He and his men were on a routine patrol in Afghanistan when the bomb detectors they were using were not going off. Things seemed quiet until he took off his backpack and set it on the ground. Once the pack came to rest, an underground bomb exploded, tearing his four limbs to shreds and leaving him devastated and on death's door. Even though he was brave and a soldier trained to survive, Sergeant Mills could no longer see the meaning of living, not until another amputee spoke to him and gave him a fresh perspective. He explained to Mills that it would take courage and that his life was worth living. The amputee gave Mills a unique gift that day by explaining everything in life is shaped by attitude.

181

From the day you're born, critical choices you make lead you on journeys down certain paths. Even as a baby, learning to crawl led you to develop essential aspects in your life, leading you to stand, walk, and, as you grew stronger, to eventually run. It is your choice on how to live after limb loss. You can forge ahead with a positive or negative outlook, it is up to you—the choice is yours to make. Having a positive outlook is something critical for life as an amputee. Life is fragile and a poor attitude can overwhelm your senses, making it even harder to reach the joy you desire. Everything is within your grasp, and the choices you make influence everything in your life. Choose who remains within your circle. Surround yourself with positive people. Choosing the right people will keep you on track and help with support moving forward. Do not let the negativity of others affect how you live and influence your progress. The right attitude involves making smart choices, which will affect your future. Luciano Pavarotti, the famous Italian opera tenor, in his autobiography, *Pavarotti, My Own Story*, spoke about the influence of his father and the choices he made. Luciano studied voice and enrolled in college, not sure whether to pursue music full on or go into teaching. One afternoon, while talking to his father, he asked, "What should I do? Should I sing or teach?" His father replied, "If you try to sit on two chairs, you will fall between them. For life, you must choose one chair." Pavarotti heeded that advice and became one of the world's greatest tenors, never regretting pursuing music as a career. Luciano later said, "Commitment is the key. Choose one chair."[2] Just as Pavarotti did, choosing how you want to live your life and having the right attitude is not only beneficial but can be a factor that carries you when things get tough. A positive attitude is a conscious choice you must make to live steadfast throughout arduous times. Learning to live as an amputee involves choosing positivity when your willpower and confidence are challenged beyond comprehension. The choice is yours and could be the significant difference between rising in life or sinking fast.

There will be times when your days may seem troublesome, lonely, and even out of sorts. Everyone experiences this, but being an amputee, these feelings crop up and seem magnified and can have a profound effect on the people around you. The mood you project, positive or negative, directly influences everyone around you. Remember, everyone, including your children, parents, partner, family, and friends, benefits from your positive attitude and demeanor. There is a responsibility being an amputee, meaning that you must do everything within your power to remain a positive influence on those around you. How we live our daily lives has a profound effect on everyone around us because your actions and words, consciously or subconsciously, possess the power to influence, heal, or hurt.

Everyone strives to control their own lives, yet the universe and the world around us are a constant reminder that no one has full control. The only things we can fully control are ourselves and our actions. You have the direct power to influence through action, which means the closer you are to people, the more significant your influence is on them. Actions truly do speak louder than words, and to others around you, your ability to depict strength, bravery, compassion, and understanding is a true daily miracle. Martin G., a double-leg above-the-knee amputee, told me he tries his best not to let negativity get him down. "I feel responsible to others to remain positive," he said. "I want to show them you can do anything you set your mind to every day." Martin's attitude conveys that affirmative actions can be a powerful weapon in showing others who you are by simply doing what you do.

Inspiration is the sister to influence, and your actions as an amputee can be an inspiration to many around you. Inspiration is found through desires and nurturing of our own unique personalities, either through creativity, music, writing, art, and heartfelt dreams and wishes. Oscar Wilde, the famous Irish poet, once said, "Be yourself; everyone else is already taken." Living as an amputee places you in a class of people that are perceived as strong and brave individuals who have endured some of the most traumatic events anyone has ever gone through. This is a powerful inspiration and truth because everyone has that special something, talent, or gift, but by exploiting what you do best inspires others around you. Remember, positive action, displaying what you are made of, and never quitting or backing down from a challenge is motivational and inspirational to so many others.

GETTING READY FOR LIFE'S BATTLE

Whether we recognize it, every one of us is equipped to face hard and difficult challenges. Author Nishan Panwar, in his book, *If Money Grew on Trees . . . Girls Would Date Monkeys*, said "You were given this life because you are strong enough to live it." He also wrote, "A beautiful life does not just happen; it is built daily by prayer, humility, sacrifice and hard work."[3] Limb loss is the ultimate test of facing adversity with something you least expected. Perhaps you believe you are not strong enough to get through it, yet there is one essential fact I want you to understand. The person who gets tested the most is usually the one who finishes the strongest and is usually the best prepared for the fight.

There isn't any doubt that losing a limb is one of the hardest events in your life and you must fight hard to get back the life you once knew. Fighting for what you want usually involves facing a degree of fear. In his book, *Rare Air / I Can't Accept Not Trying, Michael Jordan on the Pursuit of Excellence*, Michael Jordan once said, "Never say never, because limits, like fears, are often an illusion."[4]

Since the dawn of man, facing hardships and dealing with life's adversities are ingrained in our DNA. There will be days where you may not think you can make it through this traumatic time, but you are wrong—you can. Most of us, when faced with adversity, are guilty of thinking or saying to ourselves, *I can't do this, or I cannot handle this in my life; this is just way too hard.* Do everything you can to not believe or take these thoughts to heart. Helen Keller once said, "Resolve to keep happy, and your joy, and you shall form an invincible host against difficulties." Limb loss, by virtue is a "wintertime season of your life," yet as you know, after every winter — springtime always follows. This rings true in getting back to your life because your "wintertime" will hit hard mentally, physically, and emotionally. The pain and the emotions may cascade like a snowstorm, yet through your will, strength, and human spirit, your light and your newfound hope will emerge as the springtime of your life. It is there for the taking and just around the corner.

Learning the power of my thoughts after my limb loss changed the course of my life. Once I understood how my thoughts affected every area of my life, it changed the game. Your thoughts and how you react to them affect others around you, but most of all they affect how you think about yourself. Germany Kent, author of *The Hope Book*, wrote, "You become what you digest into your spirit. Whatever you think about, focus on, read about, talk about, you're going to attract more of into your life. Make sure they're all positive."[5]

Positive thinking about every aspect of your life uplifts spirit and affirms healing, which is necessary in moving forward with your life. Acceptance of your limb loss comes by loving yourself in a healthy, balanced way. In the beginning it is natural to see your limb loss negatively, but self-discovery is derived through peace and total acceptance. Prolonged negative thoughts can devastate inner growth and leave you empty and spent. To avoid this, you must start loving yourself healthily and doing everything within your power, a promise to yourself, to reach for new heights never imagined. This begins with full acceptance, and here are a few suggested steps to help with your journey of acceptance:

- Seeking help and support through peers and trusted family
- Talking to other amputees
- Joining local and national amputee groups
- Amputee roundtable group discussions
- Open talk therapy with a professional or group
- Consulting one-on-one with professionals about depression or anxiety
- Journaling
- Dieting
- Striving for self-improvement
- Reading books on resiliency, acceptance, and self-healing
- Meditation
- Transcendental meditation
- Yoga

Use whatever adaptive activities and ways that you are comfortable with that reinforce overall wellness. This is your time, and remember, doing these things does not mean that you are neglecting everyone, being self-centered, or closed off. This is merely you putting yourself first to heal physically, emotionally, and mentally. Now is the moment to do something that you haven't done before achieving new heights and long-lasting results.

Tina D., an above-the-knee amputee, lost her leg in a car accident when a drunk driver collided with her car. She and I spoke during a certified peer visit. She confessed, "I saw myself as ugly and unwanted. I did not want anyone to see me, and I wanted to crawl in a hole—and die. It wasn't without a lot of hard work, tears, and hours of self-analysis that I could think good about myself once again. However, my therapist, friends, and the peer visits taught me to think positively about myself once again. Now I know I am not ugly."

In the beginning Tina saw herself as being inadequate, broken, and not whole. I reassured her this was a normal and that she needed to understand that even though she was missing her legs, the person inside, her spirit, her heart, her desires, and her dreams were still intact. The same advice I give to you. No matter where you are in your recovery or what type of amputee you are, the same person is inside. Even though your life has changed, and even if things will have to be addressed in different ways, the person you are inside is still intact. Remember, you have only lost limb/s—not yourself—or your life.

Moving on with your new life means removing negative thoughts and replacing them with affirmative, positive thoughts about yourself. Do you like yourself, or do you feel ugly? Be honest when answering these questions. If the answer is no, you don't like yourself, you must act because it will affect your entire life. One of the hardest, yet most important things I've learned through my journey as an amputee, is to have an open and honest relationship with yourself. The connection between your thoughts and spirit is powerful, and there is an even stronger link between your attitude and how you treat others. Throughout your life with limb loss, you will be met with challenges and difficulties that can get the best of you. How you react to them, whether with anger or frustration, affects everyone around you. So if you're continually condemning yourself, it will affect, even damage relationships with your family and friends.

As an amputee, from your career to other things in your life, no matter how hard you try, you may not achieve them on your own. You may need the help of others or because of your limb loss, you may not keep the same goals.

Don't quit and never give up.

I have always been a person who goes after lofty dreams. Still, throughout the years, there were ventures I tried but failed miserably—but I never quit. I still had big dreams even after my limb loss, yet once I began my recovery, it was quickly apparent that I could not achieve those same dreams. Instead of getting down about it, I lifted myself by pursuing other dreams, ones I had placed on the back burner throughout my life. One of them being writing, which led me to write this book. The book you hold would not have been possible if it weren't for being open to following a different path. Take this time to be open to new things, develop your own path, and allow your life to take an alternative course. Embrace every new possibility until you find the one thing you desire to do more than anything else—and do it.

A POWERFUL PERSPECTIVE

Anne Frank once said, "I don't think of all the misery but the beauty that still remains."[6] This statement rings so true with many amputees. It can prove challenging to see the beauty in your life and situation. Each of us knows how we see the world and how we want to live. There are some people who see problems magnified more so than they really are. Then there are those who may see problems as mere bumps in the road and choose to see the beauty in everything in front of them. Are you one of those people? Ask yourself, where do you fit into the picture? Do you feel you still have a lot of growing to do with your limb loss? Having a powerful, influential, and healthy perspective is essential in adapting to your life as an amputee. Getting back to the things you love to do along with enjoying your family and friends is medicine for your soul. An essential aspect to living an abundant life is understanding it will be hard, but accepting and fully embracing the difficulty and working around it is the key.

By adapting your daily life around this acceptance, you will see your life blossom before your eyes. However, there may be days where you feel defeated by your circumstances. That's normal, but know you can overcome it. In society, millions of people think negatively. It appears we're all caught in an ocean of mass confusion and chaos. Many amputees lower their heads and try to get through life by having a spiritless perspective. I encourage you to take a different route. Embark on a new journey and instead explore new things, lift yourself up, meet new people, and get out and enjoy the world. Your best life is yet to come and great things are right in front of you. You, and only you, are in control of the rest of your life and have the power to make a difference. Maybe the answer for you is to help other amputees cope with their new journey. Make the difference. There is joy in helping others and committing yourself to instilling hope in others. I know firsthand—it can be contagious.

Living with limb loss is a major challenge, but you must be willing to change. It won't be easy so empower yourself by changing your perspective. When feeling hopeless, you have the power to change the negative feelings and rise above adverse circumstances. It is up to you to take the initiative and make the best of things with a positive, healthy, and hopeful perspective. However, through all this there will be times in your life that you feel you're moving backward. Still, only you can ensure your life continues to move forward, even when everything makes no sense at all. Your life will take on new meaning by adapting a powerful, life-giving, heartfelt view of living with limb loss. Remember, the best way to change things is by changing your attitude from negative to positive. Trust in knowing there will be unanswered questions and days where your problems seem gargantuan and out of control, but choosing to see the good in these circumstances is the answer to living the best life possible.

BEING A PART OF AMPUTEES WORLDWIDE

The one most essential aspect I have learned as an amputee is that every amputee, young or old, famous or not, has a definitive chance to change their lives and impact the lives of others around them.

And you do, too.

Many famous amputees around the world (some you may not have even known were amputees) have affected many people's lives. Unfortunately, the media does not shed much light on amputees. Instead, increased awareness and sympathy have grown for various mental illnesses; however, amputation continues to have something of a darker, unrecognized public stigma. There seems to be an unfortunate "embarrassment aspect" that is often associated with amputation despite the ever-increasing steps toward accommodating people with physical disabilities, such as handicapped-accessible stalls, priority seating on airplanes, and exterior ramps built at entranceways of many buildings. Still, the media has primarily kept limb loss under wraps. For example, most people don't know that these past and present celebrities were (or are) amputees:

Jerry Garcia: Legendary guitarist for The Grateful Dead, who lost his middle finger in a camping accident at age four.

Rahm Emanuel: Former mayor of Chicago and chief of staff for President Obama, who lost his finger in an accident.

Bethany Hamilton: Champion surfer who lost her arm in a shark attack.

Ella Fitzgerald: Renowned jazz singer who had both legs amputated because of diabetes.

Aimee Mullins: Athlete, actress, and fashion model born with fibular hemimelia (a condition in which the individual is missing fibula bones) that resulted in the amputation of both her legs below the knees.

Bill Veeck: Owner of three Major League Baseball teams who lost his leg in World War II.

Rick Allen: The Def Leppard drummer who lost his left arm in a car accident.

Heather Mills: British media personality and model who lost the bottom half of her leg below the knee in a traffic accident.

Waylon Jennings: Singer/songwriter whose foot was amputated because of diabetes.

Zsa Zsa Gabor: Actress whose leg was amputated because of an infection.

Tony Iommi: Black Sabbath guitarist who lost the tips of his fingers in a machinery accident at a young age.

James Doohan: Famed "Scotty" of *Star Trek* had one of his middle fingers shot off during World War II.

Cole Porter: Iconic composer who suffered from osteomyelitis, a bone disease that ultimately led to the loss of his left leg.

Ron Santo: Major League Baseball player for the Chicago Cubs and Hall of Famer who had the lower half of both legs amputated because of diabetes.

Whether these individuals preferred to keep their respective amputations private or the media concealed them because of perceived stigmas associated with them is unknown.

For most of us strength is the physical ability to lift, push, or pull, and as an amputee, physical strength is essential to your new amputee life; however, strength can mean something different entirely. Strength, as an amputee, can be found in being mentally and emotionally able to handle what life throws at you. Being strong can also mean being strong of mind and understanding when to react, or not, to circumstances in your life. Strength is derived from overcoming immense obstacles and facing brutally hard challenges by learning how to overpower them in your own unique way, which is one of the first significant signs of inner strength, which can be more important and even stronger than outer strength. Building physical strength is difficult, but it can be accomplished through exercise, lifting heavy weights or objects, and simple movement. Inner strength is built in the same way, only through unforeseen lifting and pulling of the present heavy burdens on our hearts, mind, and soul.

Managing your life as an amputee is personal, a unique event—a situation where you will respond to things differently than others. Everyone manages their lives differently. Here are a few ways to ensure your life is the best it can be:

- Manage stress by being assertive and avoiding being aggressive.
- Do your best to plan ahead.
- Don't procrastinate. Address everything head-on.
- Think everything through. Set yourself up for the best outcome by making this part of your routine.
- Stay positive, and never let negativity bring you down.
- Do your best to get a good night's sleep.
- Give yourself "me" time through meditation and other relaxation techniques.
- Read quietly, which can relieve stress.
- Meet with like-minded amputees.
- Always keep safety at the forefront.
- Communicate openly.
- Express appreciation and gratitude toward others.
- Stay vigilant and work hard in all that you do.
- Be humble.
- Never quit.

Limb loss is not a race, and it is best to not compare yourself to others and their efforts. However, you may find inspiration in being around other amputees who can uplift, provide guidance, and help you strengthen your mind and spirit. The Amputee Coalition (www.

amputee-coaltion.org) offers peer support, answers questions, and has people there who will listen when you just need someone to talk to. They can pair you with amputees who have the same limb loss as you. No matter how strong you are, every one of us needs advice and support of others. Reach out to professionals, family, or seek peer support to help you through any troublesome times in your life. Plus, admitting to one's self that you need help is a sign of inner strength, even if it doesn't feel like it.

However, you may be the person who finds strength in being alone and thrives in having time to think things through by yourself. Some people need quiet and solitude to gather their thoughts, and if so, it may be hard for others around you to understand what you are you going through. It is healthy to step back and take the time to reflect on how you should proceed with your life. There isn't a right or wrong way to gain inner strength. So stay strong and be true to yourself because you're the one living your life, and no one can live it for you.

Living life as an amputee will have immense highs and drastic lows. Remember, there isn't anything wrong with failing; the key is you must pick yourself back up—and never quit. Be strong, dig deep to find your unique power, and use the power potency to propel your life forward. The only limitations you have are the ones you place on yourself. Limb loss, though unwanted or unexpected, will undoubtedly reshape your life. Maybe you can't see it yet, but hang in there because it will. Your limb loss may incredibly save your life by setting you on a trajectory you never expected. I encourage you to embrace the newness of the unforeseen. Embrace everything about being an amputee; face every challenge with the utmost perseverance and unbridled tenacity to overcome any obstacle. We are given free will, and how you choose to live your life from this point forward is entirely up to you.

Surround yourself with people and friends that encourage you. Choose people who allow you to sustain yourself and keep your spirits lifted. Everyone in our lives realizes that they must live with the repercussions of their actions, and it is you whose reflection is in the mirror. Living with limb loss will test who you are and what you are made of, so take advantage, explore the possibilities of where you envision your life. What is that you want to do with your life? What dreams do you have that you want to achieve? Imagine yourself accomplishing everything you've ever dreamed of. Now it is your time to shine.

Eleanor Roosevelt once said, "No one can make you feel inferior without your permission."[7] With limb loss you have the power to control every aspect of your life, so do not allow feelings of inferiority to crop up and keep you from achieving your goals. Use the power within to change your thoughts, perceptions, and dreams.

It is only through determination and a strong mindset that you can make a difference. Be strong in mind, willful in spirit, and remind yourself never to give up. Although there will be days where quitting seems like the answer, remember that it shouldn't be an option. Quitting is never the answer because you will be only giving up on yourself. Losing a limb takes vast amounts of courage and strength to live a life of meaning and great conviction. Limb loss is a real-life story, a genuine display of you conquering the impossible through unrelenting human courage. Living with limb loss isn't the end of your life, nor is it considered a death. It is a beginning, a restart of a new life, a rebirth bringing opportunity to excel in greatness that you never expected.

Throughout your limb loss journey you will discover new ways, perspectives, and life-altering aspects about yourself that you never realized. You will soon encounter circumstances that will push you harder than anything before, but living with limb loss will be the adventure of your lifetime, achieved by pushing yourself to reach new heights and destinations never dreamed. What your heart is saying should remain the beacon to where your life is headed and what you want to do with your life. Charles Dickens once wrote, "The most important thing in life is to stop saying 'I wish' and start saying 'I will.' Consider nothing impossible, then treat possibilities as probabilities."

Embrace this chance and strive for victory over everything in your life. This is your unique stance, a rare lightning strike moment to turn your life into a spectacular display of the human spirit. Seize the opportunity to let your perseverance shine and make your actions speak louder than any single word. Learn to live fully, filling your soul with unparalleled beauty and wholesomeness by showing the world your unbridled spirit through sheer perseverance, strength, and action toward yourself and others. Go after your dreams with vigor and never let anyone or anything stop or stand in your way. And most importantly, never forget to love yourself and others because by doing so you can make anything impossible genuinely possible. Limb loss life is your personal journey, a victory, a celebration, and your time to show the world that you are AMPOSSIBLE!

Notes

CHAPTER 1

1. K. Ziegler-Graham, E. J. MacKenzie, P. L. Ephraim, T. G. Travison, and R. Brookmeyer, "Estimating the Prevalence of Limb Loss in the United States" 2005 to 2050, *Archives of Physical Medicine and Rehabilitation* 89, no. 3 (2008): 422–29.

2. Centers for Disease Control and Prevention, "National Diabetes Statistics Report," 2020. Atlanta, GA: Centers for Disease Control and Prevention, U.S. Dept. of Health and Human Services; 2020. https://www.cdc.gov/diabetes/pdfs/data/statistics/national-diabetes-statistics-report.pdf

3. Centers for Disease Control and Prevention, "National Diabetes Statistics Report," 2020. Atlanta, GA: Centers for Disease Control and Prevention, U.S. Dept. of Health and Human Services; 2020. https://www.cdc.gov/diabetes/pdfs/data/statistics/national-diabetes-statistics-report.pdf

4. Centers for Disease Control and Prevention, "DC Report Finds Large Decline in Lower-Limb Amputations among U.S. Adults with Diagnosed Diabetes," 2012. Centers for Disease Control and Prevention, U.S. Dept of Health and Human Services; 2020. https://www.cdc.gov/media/releases/2012/p0124_lower_limb.html

5. K. Ziegler-Graham et al., "Estimating the Prevalence," 422–29.

6. National Cancer Institute, "Cancer Statistics," last modified September 25, 2020, https://www.cancer.gov/about-cancer/understanding/statistics.

7. Statistics adapted from the American Cancer Society's publication, "Cancer Facts & Figures 2020," January 2020, https://www.cancer.net/cancer-types/bone-cancer/statistics.

8. L. C. Trautwein, D. G. Smith, and F. P. Rivera, "Pediatric amputation injuries: etiology, cost and outcome," *The Journal of Trauma* 41 (1996):831–38. R. Loder, "Demographics of traumatic amputations in children. Implications

for prevention strategies," *The American Journal of Bone and Joint Surgery*, 86-A(5) (May 2004): 923–28. https://www.amputee-coalition.org/resources/amputations-in-childhood/

9. John E. Hangar, "J. E. Hanger Lost His Leg But Not His Ingenuity," Civil War Profiles, last modified March, 16, 2013, https://www.civilwarprofiles.com/j-e-hanger-lost-his-leg-but-not-ingenuity/.

10. Hannah Fisher, "A Guide to U.S. Military Casualty Statistics: Operation Freedom's Sentinel, Operation Inherent Resolve, Operation New Dawn, Operation Iraqi Freedom, and Operation Enduring Freedom." Hannah Fischer Information Research Specialist, August 7, 2015, https://fas.org/sgp/crs/natsec/RS22452.pdf.

11. Hannah Fisher, "A Guide to U.S. Military Casualty Statistics: Operation New Dawn, Operation Iraqi Freedom, and Operation Enduring Freedom (by Hannah Fischer, Congressional Research Service), (pdf)_http://www.allgov.com/news/top-stories/leftovers-from-afghanistan-and-iraq-wars-1558-amputations-7224-severe-brain-injuries-118829-post-traumatic-stress-disorders-140303?news=852580.

12. Mayo Clinic, "Buerger's Disease: Risk Factors External Icon," 2019 Feb, https://www.cdc.gov/tobacco/campaign/tips/diseases/buergers-disease.html.

CHAPTER SEVEN

1. Bielefeld University, "Phantom Sensations: When the Sense of Touch Deceives." ScienceDaily. www.sciencedaily.com/releases/2019/06/190614111929.htm (accessed December 22, 2020).

2. Bielefeld University, "Phantom Sensations."

CHAPTER 8

1. Daniel H. Wilson, *Robopocalypse*. New York: Doubleday, 2011.

CHAPTER 9

1. Helen Keller Quotes. Goodreads by Amazon. https://www.goodreads.com/author/quotes/7275.Helen_Keller. December 27, 2020.

2. S. Forward, *Toxic Parents: Overcoming Their Hurtful Legacy and Reclaiming Your Life* (New York: Bantam). Reprint edition (December 15, 2009).
3. Mark Twain quotes. A–Z Quotes. https://www.azquotes.com/author/14883-Mark_Twain, December 27, 2020.
4. Thomas C. Weiss, "Addiction and Substance Abuse among Persons with Disabilities," Electronic Publication Date: 2013-07-22. Last Revised Date: 2020-11-12. https://www.disabled-world.com/medical/pharmaceutical/addiction/serious.php.
5. Richard Bach, *Illusions: The Adventures of a Reluctant Messiah* (New York: Arrow Books, 1977).

CHAPTER 10

1. J. K. Rowling quotes, Good Reads by Amazon: https://www.goodreads.com/quotes/67454-understanding-is-the-first-step-to-acceptance-and-only-with.

CHAPTER 11

1. Peggy Chenowerth, *Becoming Comfortable with Sex and Intimacy After a Limb Amputation.* https://themighty.com/2016/10/sex-and-intimacy-after-limb-amputation/.
2. Aimee Mullins. "The Inspirational Aimee Mullins." *Huffington Post*, Published 01/05/2011 12:59 pm ET Updated Dec 06, 2017.

CHAPTER 12

1. Jim Abbott, Inspiring Quotes, 2020. https://www.inspiringquotes.us/author/7688-jim-abbott.
2. Richelle E. Goodrich. *Making Wishes: Quotes, Thoughts, and a Little Poetry for Every Day of the Year.* August 6, 2015.
3. Karen Calhoun, "Amputee Coalition and Össur Partner to Improve the Well Being of amputees." Yahoo News. http://www.yahoo.com/news/.

CHAPTER 13

1. Chris Boulias, Ben Meikle, Tim Pauley, and Michael Devlin, "Return to Driving After Lower-Extremity Amputation," *Archives of Physical Medicine and Rehabilitation*, Volume 87, Issue 9,2006, Pages 1183-1188, ISSN 0003-9993, https://doi.org/10.1016/j.apmr.2006.06.001. (http://www.sciencedirect.com/science/article/pii/S0003999306005211).

2. "Adapted Vehicles," Article: National Highway and Traffic Safety Board, Published Date Unknown. https://www.nhtsa.gov/road-safety/drivers-disabilities.

CHAPTER 14

1. World Health Organization, *Violence against Adults and Children with Disabilities*. Published July 2012: https://www.who.int/disabilities/violence/en/.

2. *Violence against Adults and Children with Disabilities*.

3. Jeff Cooper, *Principles of Personal Defense*. Paladin Press; Revised edition (January 1, 2006).

CHAPTER 15

1. Emily's Quotes. H.W Arnold. 2020, https://emilysquotes.com/the-worst-bankruptcy-in-the-world-is-the-person-who-has-lost-his-enthusiasm/.

2. David U. Himmelstein, Robert M. Lawless, Deborah Thorne, Pamela Foohey, and Steffie Woolhandler, "Medical Bankruptcy: Still Common Despite the Affordable Care Act," *American Journal of Public Health* 109: 431–33. https://doi.org/10.2105/AJPH.2018.304901.

3. Essential C.S. Lewis Quotes. Published May 2018 http://essentialcslewis.com/2015/08/29/hardships-often-prepare-ordinary-people/.

4. Malcolm Gladwell, *Blink*, Back Bay Books; Annotated edition (April 3, 2007).

CHAPTER 16

1. *The Dollar Store Diet,* University of Nevada, Las Vegas. Published February 2019. https://www.unlv.edu/news/article/dollar-store-diet-produce-quality-matches-traditional-chains.

CHAPTER 18

1. Travis Mills, *Travis—A Soldier's Story.* Fotolanthropy Production:2020: http://travisthemovie.com/.
2. Luciano Pavarotti, *Pavarotti, My Own Story*, Doubleday, 1981.
3. Nishan Panwar, *If Money Grew on Trees...Girls Would Date Monkeys.* CreateSpace Independent Publishing Platform (November 16, 2014).
4. Jordan, Michael. *Rare Air / I Can't Accept Not Trying, Michael Jordan on the Pursuit of Excellence,* Rare Air Ltd (January 1, 1994).
5. Germany Kent, *The Hope Book*; Star Stone Press. March 10, 2015.
6. Anne Frank. *The Diary of a Young Girl.* Bantam; Reissue edition (June 1, 1993).
7. Eleanor Roosevelt, Brainy Quote LLC. https://www.brainyquote.com/quotes/eleanor_roosevelt_161321.

Bibliography

Abbott, Jim. 2020. Inspiring Quotes. https://www.inspiringquotes.us/author/7688-jim-abbott.

American Journal of Public Health 109, 431_433, https://doi.org/10.2105/AJPH.2018.304901.

Arnold. W. H. 2020. *Emily's Quotes*. Published 2020, https://emilysquotes.com/the-worst-bankruptcy-in-the-world-is-the-person-who-has-lost-his-enthusiasm/.

Bach, Richard. 1989. *Illusions: The Adventures of a Reluctant Messiah*. New York: Dell.

Bielefeld University. "Phantom Sensations: When the Sense of Touch Deceives." ScienceDaily. www.sciencedaily.com/releases/2019/06/190614111929.htm (accessed December 22, 2020).

Boulias, Chris, et al. 2006. "Return to Driving After Lower-Extremity Amputation." *Archives of Physical Medicine and Rehabilitation*, Volume 87, Issue 9, 2006, 1183–88, https://doi.org/10.1016/j.apmr.2006.06.001. (http://www.sciencedirect.com/science/article/pii/S0003999306005211).

Breuss, Adolf. 1995. *The Bruess Cancer Cure*. New York: Bantam.

Calhoun, Karen. 2017. "Amputee Coalition and Ossur Partner to Improve the Well Being of Amputees." Yahoo News. http://www.yahoo.com/news/ Published October 2017.

Chenowerth, Peggy. "Becoming Comfortable With Sex and Intimacy After a Limb Amputation." https://themighty.com/2016/10/sex-and-intimacy-after-limb-amputation/.

Cooper, Jeff. 2006. *Principles of Personal Defense*. Paladin Press.

Forword, Susan. 2009. *Toxic Parents: Overcoming Their Hurtful Legacy and Reclaiming Your Life*. New York: Bantam.

Frank, Anne. 1993. *The Diary of a Young Girl*. Bantam; Reissue edition (June 1, 1993).

Gladwell, Malcolm. 2007. *Blink*. Back Bay Books.

Goodrich, Richelle E. 2015. *Making Wishes: Quotes, Thoughts, & a Little Poetry for Every Day of the Year.* CreateSpace Independent Publishing.

Gregory, Rebekah. 2017. *Taking Back My Life: My Story of Faith, Determination, and Surviving the Boston Marathon Bombing.* Ada, MIL Revell.

Himmelstein, David et al. 2019. *Medical Bankruptcy: Still Common Despite the Affordable Care Act.*

Jordan, Michael. 1994. *Rare Air / I Can't Accept Not Trying, Michael Jordan on the Pursuit of Excellence.* Rare Air Ltd.

Kent, Germany. 2015. *The Hope Book.* Star Stone Press.

Kirkup, John. 2006. *History of Limb Amputation.* New York: Springer.

Krajbich, Joseph Ivan et al. 2018. *Atlas of Amputations and Limb Deficiencies* (4th ed.). New York: Wolters Kluwer.

Kubler-Ross, Elizabeth. 2014. *On Death and Dying.* New York: Scribner.

Laphie, Leah. Cram.com. 2020. https://www.cram.com/essay/Life-Lesson-In-The-American-Idol-By/P3YRT653UZ3Q https://www.cram.com/essay/Life-Lesson-In-The-American-Idol-By/P3YRT653UZ3Q.

Lewis, C. S. 2009. *A Grief Observed.* New York: HarperOne.

———. 2018. *Essential C.S. Lewis Quotes:* Published May 2018. http://essentialcslewis.com/2015/08/29/hardships-often-prepare-ordinary-people/.

Mark Twain quotes. https://www.azquotes.com/author/14883-Mark_Twain. December 27, 2020.

Mills, Travis. 2020. *Travis- A Soldier's Story.* Fotolanthropy Production. http://travisthemovie.com/.

Malchow, Dee. 2016. *Alive & Whole: Amputation: Emotional Recovery.* CreateSpace Independent Publishing.

Mullins, Aimee. 2017. *The Inspirational Aimee Mullins:* Huffington Post. Published 01/05/2011. Updated Dec 06, 2017.

Murphy, Douglas. 2014. *Fundamentals of Amputation Care and Prosthetics.* New York: Springer.

Murray, Craig. 2009. *Amputation, Prosthesis Use, Phantom Sensations.* New York: Springer.

National Highway and Traffic Safety Board. 2015. *Adapted Vehicles:* Published Date- Unknown. https://www.nhtsa.gov/road-safety/drivers-disabilities

Panwar, Nishan. 2014. *If Money Grew on Trees...Girls Would Date Monkeys.* CreateSpace Independent Publishing Platform.

Pavarotti, Luciano. 1981. *Pavarotti, My Own Story.* New York: Doubleday.

Rowling, J. K. 2020. J.K Rowling Quotes, Good Reads by Amazon: https://www.goodreads.com/quotes/67454-understanding-is-the-first-step-to-acceptance-and-only-with.

Rheinstein, John. 2016. *Atlas of Amputations and Limb Deficiencies* (4th ed.), Hangar Clinic.

Roosevelt, Eleanor. 2020. Brainy Quote LLC. https://www.brainyquote.com/quotes/eleanor_roosevelt_161321

Rosenberger, Gracie. 2018. "Living with Amputation: Gracie Rosenberger's Story." https://www.webmd.com/women/features/living-with-amputation-gracie-rosenbergers-story#1

Wallace, Carol. 1995. *Challenged by Amputation: Embracing a New Life*. Inclusion Concepts Publishing House.

Weiss. C. Thomas. 2013. *Addiction and Substance Abuse Among Persons with Disabilities*. Source: https://www.disabled-world.com/medical/pharmaceutical/addiction/serious.php

Wilson, Daniel H. 2011. *Robopocalypse*. New York: Doubleday.

World Health Organization. 2012. *Violence against Adults and Children with Disabilities*: https://www.who.int/disabilities/violence/en/

Index

Abbott, Jim, 125
above knee amputation, 23, 84; left, 137
acceptance, 96–97, 100, 180; by children, 110–11; by family members, 110–11; in grief, 91; of limb loss, 26–27, 77, 185; of prosthetic limb, 131–33
acetaminophen, 67
activities of daily living, 31–32, 103; modifications to, 58–59
acupuncture, 68
ADA. *See* Americans with Disabilities Act
adaptive prosthetic technology, 84
Addair, George, 154
addiction: alcohol, 94, 97, 99; drug, 97–98; medication, 67–68; recovery, 97
adventitious bursae, 48–49
adversity, 184
alcohol dependency, 94, 97, 99
Alive & Whole, 40
Allen, Rick, 189
allergic reaction, 52–53
American Journal of Public Health, 153
American Red Cross, 57–58
Americans with Disabilities Act (ADA), 158–59, 162

amputation: before, 9–35; below knee, 4, 23; bilateral, 138; bilateral arms/hands, 139–41; bilateral legs/feet, 138; cancer and, 12–15, 21, 44; causes for, 11–18; complications after, 47–53; congenital, 13, 15–16, 113; death or, 4; diabetes and, 12–14; disclosure of, 159; effects of, 6; facing your, 1–8; of hand, finger, or arms, 139; above knee, 23, 84, 137; left-sided, 136, 137; of little toe, 3; lower extremity/limb, 14, 23, 33, 39, 44–45, 50–51, 55, 61–62, 79, 127–29; major, 17; multiple limb, 39, 56; nontraumatic, 12, 48; nurses and, 30–31; occupational therapist and, 31–32; PAD and, 12, 14; pain after, 52; physical recovery after, 37–85; physical therapist and, 31; podiatrist and, 33; primary care physician and, 30; prosthetist and, 22, 32–33, 59, 83, 130–31, 163; psychologist and, 34–35; quadruple, 181; reality of, 20; recovery, 21; rehabilitation specialist and, 32; right-sided, 136, 137; as routine procedure, 5;

203

About the Author

Jeffrey Allen Mangus is president of LIMB LOSS LIFE LLC and the CEO of Ghostwriting USA. He has survived three life-threatening heart attacks, a quintuple heart bypass, five amputations, and sepsis.

Pushing himself through recovery after losing his left leg below the knee, Jeffrey now speaks to other amputees around the world as a Certified Peer Visitor (CPV) through the Amputee Coalition of America. He is currently active in CPV limb loss support and speaks with many amputees across the United States upon request.

He has ghostwritten numerous award-winning business books for many independent businesspeople, CEOs, and leaders around the globe.

CPSIA information can be obtained
at www.ICGtesting.com
Printed in the USA
BVHW071557090821
614005BV00002B/2

9 781538 141878